THE
NUTRITIONAL
COST OF DRUGS

**A Guide to Maintaining Good Nutrition
While Using Prescription and
Over-the-Counter Drugs,** Second Edition

Ross Pelton, R.Ph., Ph.D., C.C.N.

James B. LaValle, R.Ph., N.M.D., C.C.N.

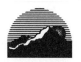

Morton Publishing Company
925 West Kenyon Avenue, Unit 12
Englewood, CO 80110
www.morton-pub.com

BOOK TEAM

Publisher	Douglas N. Morton
Project Manager	Dona Mendoza
Copy Editor	Carolyn Acheson
Cover & Design	Bob Schram, Bookends
Composition	International Typesetting & Composition

A NOTE TO READERS

Readers may find that a drug they are taking is not mentioned in this reference book. In such cases, no studies have been conducted to evaluate whether the drug causes nutrient depletion, which is the unfortunate case with many of the newer drugs on the market. In a future edition of this book, we plan to include a complete index of all available drugs, and in that index we will include new drugs that have been released but are not listed, with the indication "none" for those on which no studies on nutrient depletions have been conducted yet.

CONTENTS

FOREWORD v
INTRODUCTION vii
How to Use This Book vii
Scientific Basis.......................viii
A Message About Health............ix
The Safety of Nutritional
Supplements..........................x

PART I: QUICK REFERENCE GUIDE
TO NUTRIENTIONAL LOSSES 3

PART II: DRUGS AND THEIR EFFECTS
ON NUTRITION..........................25

Antacids..............................26
Magnesium/Aluminum
Hydroxide Antacids.............26
Sodium Bicarbonate
Antacids.........................26

Anti-Anxiety Agents:
Benzodiazepines......................27
Diazepam and Alprazolam......27

Antibiotics 27
Antibiotics To Treat
Tuberculosis...................29
Aminogylcosides 33
Antimalarial Antibiotics..........33
Penicillin Antibiotics 34
Tetracycline Antibiotics...........34
Trimethoprim.......................35

Anticonvulsants 35
Barbiturates 35
Phenytoin............................38
Carbamazepine 41
Primidone 43
Valproic Acid.......................45

Antidiabetic Drugs...................46
Sulfonylureas 46
Biguanides...........................46

Antifungals: Amphotericin B 48

Antihistamines: Hydroxyzine......48

Anti-Inflammatory Drugs 49
Corticosteroids......................49
Salicylates (Aspirin)................52
Sulfasalazine 53
Indomethacin 53
Other Non-Steroidal
Anti-Inflammatory Drugs
(NSAIDs) 53

Anti-Parkinson's Disease
Drug: Levodopa....................54

Antiprotozoals: Pentamidine........55

Antiviral Drugs......................55
Reverse Transcriptase
Inhibitors: Zidovudine (AZT)
and Related Drugs 55
Foscarnet 56

Bronchodilators 56
Theophylline 56
Beta$_2$ Adrenergic Agonists.......57

Cardiovascular Drugs 57
ACE Inhibitors......................58
Beta-blockers 58
Calcium Channel Blockers:
Nifedipine and Verapamil.....59
Cardiac Glycosides:
Digoxin...........................59
Centrally Acting
Antihypertensive Agents:
Clonidine and Methyldopa....60
Hydralazine-containing
Vasodilators 60
Loop Diuretics 61
Potassium-sparing Diuretics....63
Thiazide Diuretics..................64

Chemotherapy Drugs.................65

Cholesterol-Lowering Drugs 66
  HMG-CoA Reductase
    Inhibitors (the Statins) 66
  Bile Acid Sequestrants.............66
  The Fibrates 67
  Gemfibrozil 68

Electrolyte Replacement:
Timed-Release Potassium
Chloride.....................................68

Female Hormones......................69
  Oral Contraceptives................69
  Estrogen Replacement
    Therapy 73

Gout Medications: Colchicine 75

Laxatives 76
  Laxatives Containing
    Mineral Oil 76
  Bisacodyl................................76
  Phosphate Enemas 77

Psychotherapeutic Drugs 77
  Tricyclic Antidepressants.........77
  Phenothiazines 78
  Monoamine Oxidase Inhibitors
    (MAOIs) (Phenelzine
    and Haloperidol) 78
  Lithium 79
  Selective Serotonin Reuptake
    Inhibitors (SSRIs)..................79

Steroids (Anabolic) 79

Thyroid Medications 80

Ulcer Medications 80
  H-2 Blockers...........................81
  Proton Pump Inhibitors 82

Miscellaneous Drugs....................83
  Methotrexate 83
  Penicillamine..........................84
  EDTA.....................................85
  Ritodrine.................................85

PART III: NUTRIENT REVIEWS 89
  Beta-Carotene 90
  Bifidobacteria Bifidum
    (bifidus) 91
  Biotin 92
  Boron 94
  Calcium 95

Carnitine..................................98
Chloride...................................99
Choline 100
Chromium 102
Coenzyme Q10 104
Copper...................................106
Fluoride 108
Folic Acid (Folacin)...............110
Inositol...................................113
Iodine.....................................114
Iron...116
Lactobacillus Acidophilus 118
Magnesium 120
Manganese.............................123
Melatonin 125
Molybdenum 126
Nickel 127
Phosphorus 129
Potassium...............................131
S-Adenosyl Methionine
  (SAMe) 132
Selenium 134
Silicon 136
Sodium...................................138
Sulfur 139
Vanadium 140
Vitamin A (Retinol) 142
Vitamin B_1 (Thiamin)...........144
Vitamin B_2 (Riboflavin) 146
Vitamin B_3 (Niacin) 148
Vitamin B_5 (Pantothenic
  Acid) 150
Vitamin B_6 (Pyridoxine) 151
Vitamin B_{12}
  (Cyanocobalamin)...............154
Vitamin C (Ascorbic Acid)....156
Vitamin D (Calciferol) 159
Vitamin E (Alpha
  Tocopherol).........................161
Vitamin K 164
Zinc 165

PART IV: BRAND NAMES/
GENERIC NAMES....................171

GLOSSARY 181
APPENDIX......................................195
INDEX..201

FOREWORD

OVER THE LAST DECADE or more, the importance of a healthy diet, including the wise use of vitamins and minerals, has received much emphasis and publicity. Despite our best efforts to stay well, though, prescription or non-prescription drugs are necessary from time to time. And for some of us, circumstances necessitate the continuous use of one or more non-prescription drugs.

Unfortunately, easily accessible and useful information about the interactions between prescription drugs and nutrients in the body has been lacking. The "warnings" we occasionally receive about vitamin or mineral use from drug prescribers are often overly broad or not well supported. Even worse, many of us have come to realize that information about drugs and nutrients from government agencies is not always reliable.

That's why *The Nutritional Cost of Drugs* is a uniquely valuable book. In this reference, Ross Pelton and Jim LaValle have assembled documented information that the typical prescription and over-the-counter drug user might find useful to avoid hazardous drug-nutrient interactions and take nutritional measures to correct drug-induced nutritional deficiencies. Best of all, this book is an easy-to-understand "primer" on the uses of the vitamins and minerals in the body.

Now that you have this uniquely valuable resource, why not show it to your doctor? You also might mention that a "professional" version is available in an easy-to-use handbook form, *The Drug-induced Nutrient Depletion Handbook, second edition* (2003) by Ross Pelton, James B. LaValle, Ernest B. Hawkins, and Daniel L. Krinsky.*

Jonathan V. Wright, M.D.
Medical Director, Tahoma Clinic Kent, Washington

Dr. Wright is a graduate of Harvard University and the University of Michigan Medical School. He has practiced nutritional and natural medicine at the Tahoma Clinic, in Kent, Washington, since 1973. His several books, including the recent best-selling Natural Hormone Replacement for Women Over 45, *have sold more than 750,000 copies. He and his colleague, Alan R. Gaby, M.D., teach nationally respected seminars in nutritional medicine for health care professionals.*

---

*Published by Lexi-Comp, Inc., 1100 Terex Road, Hudson, OH 44236, www.lexi.com.

INTRODUCTION

THE NUTRITIONAL COST OF DRUGS is a reference book for those who are taking prescription or over-the-counter drugs, as related to the nutrients those drugs deplete within the body. The medical term — *drug-induced nutrient depletion* — has become a hot new health topic. Unlike many topics that are fads that come and go, drug-induced nutrient depletions is not a fad. It is moving to center stage because it is of vital significance to health professionals as well as the general public. The information in this book will help those who take medications regularly to learn how to prevent or overcome drug-induced nutrient depletion and maintain good nutrition.

Studies documenting that many commonly prescribed drugs cause the depletion of one or more nutrients have been appearing in the peer-reviewed scientific literature for decades. But this information has not received the publicity and attention it deserves, until now.

This book covers over 1,000 drugs that can cause the depletion of nutrients in humans. Most of the major categories of drugs (such as oral contraceptives, antacids, antibiotics, and cardiovascular drugs) cause nutrient depletions. In a survey of the top 200 drugs dispensed in 2002, 16 of the top 20 drugs have a potential for a drug/nutrient interaction.[1] This is a problem that affects millions of people.

Many of the side effects from drugs actually may be attributable to nutrient depletions caused by the drugs when taken over time. Now that this information has been brought to light, health professionals have a professional responsibility to become knowledgeable about drug-induced nutrient depletions so they can counsel patients and customers accordingly. In reality, doctors and pharmacists often are too busy to dispense all the information you need. This book is designed to get this information into your hands as, ultimately, your health is your responsibility.

HOW TO USE THIS BOOK

This book has been organized and cross-referenced so readers can easily locate information about drugs, nutrients, and the health problems associated with specific nutrient losses. It is organized into the following parts:

■ PART I: QUICK REFERENCE CHART

This chart presents an overview of the drugs that cause the loss of nutrients. It is a brief guide to Part II, a synopsis of the information presented in that part.

■ PART II: DRUGS AND THEIR EFFECTS ON NUTRITION

This part provides a more detailed discussion of the drugs that cause nutrient losses and the potential health problems that can develop from these losses. It also provides information on sales of individual drugs or drug categories, including the sales volume and ranking in the United States for 2002, based on the annual survey of prescription drugs conducted by IMS Health.[2]

■ PART III: NUTRIENT REVIEWS

In this part, the role of each nutrient is profiled in detail, along with a listing of generic drugs that can deplete that nutrient. (The brand names of drugs are listed in Part IV.) Part III also summarizes the symptoms and causes of nutrient depletion to help you determine if your symptoms or health problems might be related to a deficiency of that nutrient. The reviews give an overview of each nutrient, information about the nutrient's biological functions and effects, side effects and toxicity, dosages, and dietary sources.

■ PART IV: BRAND NAMES / GENERIC NAMES

This part lists the brand name and associated generic name for drugs that are on the market.

SCIENTIFIC BASIS

The appendix give scientific basis for the nutrient depletions associated with the generic drugs included in this reference book. The following criteria were applied:

SB1: The most common rationale for including a drug in this book; indicates that the scientific studies reporting a nutrient depletion(s) were conducted using this specific drug.

SB2: Indicates that studies from drugs in the same pharmacological class have reported nutrient depletions. For example, assume that no studies have reported that drug X has depleted any nutrients. Nevertheless, if studies have reported that other drugs in the same pharmacological class have caused nutrient depletions, it can be assumed that drug X could deplete the same nutrients.

SB3: Refers to a drug that works the same way as another drug that is known to cause a nutrient depletion (both drugs have the same mechanism of action.)

SB4: Designates drugs for which there is inferred or indirect evidence of depletion based on disruption of physiological processes. An example is when chemotherapy drugs or antibiotics disrupt the normal functioning of the gastrointestinal tract.

It would be virtually impossible to track down every study that has been published on the wide range of drugs included in this book. Nevertheless, we believe we have located most of the studies that have been published on drug-induced nutrient depletions, and we have attempted to provide balance by factoring in negative or conflicting studies where they exist. Most of our database research was conducted online on Medline, which contains most recognized medical journals.

For space and cost reasons, a listing of the scientific studies we researched is not included in this book. Our primary goal in this documentation is to verify to health professionals and the general public that a large and credible body of scientific research has reported and documented drug-induced nutrient depletions.

In developing this book, we are not suggesting that drug-induced nutrient deficiencies are the primary source of people's medical problems. Conditions such as high stress, environmental pollution, poor nutrition, and many other factors can contribute to health problems. When people take medications that create additional nutrient losses, however, this may be the proverbial straw that breaks the camel's back. Nutrient depletions can have a negative effect on digestion, metabolism, detoxification, and other facets of metabolic function, ultimately disrupting an individual's immune system and overall health.

We suspect that the problem of drug-induced nutrient depletions is much larger and more widespread than is reported in this book. In many cases, a drug's effect on various nutrients has simply not been studied yet. Funding for such studies is difficult to come by, but we hope the evidence presented in this book will stimulate more research in this area and require rigorous testing before approval of new drugs. Gaining insight into nutrient depletions caused by drugs, we hope, will enable us to reduce symptoms and side effects of drugs, allowing for improved quality of care.

A MESSAGE ABOUT HEALTH

A number of years ago we saw one of Ashleigh Brilliant's humorous postcards that stated, "Life is the only game in which the object of the game is to learn the rules."[3] That little statement made a strong impression on us, as a serious statement about health and life. When you purchase a new car or any appliance, you receive with it a detailed operating manual with instructions on how to care for it, keep it running smoothly, and trouble-shoot problems. We come into life with an amazingly complex, wonderful machine called the human body, which has no operating manual. Unfortunately, many people don't bother to take care of the body until it starts to break down. If we learn some of the simple, basic fundamental rules of health, it ultimately will make the Game of Life much longer and more enjoyable.

Ever since their inception many years ago, standards such as Recommended Dietary Allowance (RDAs) have been promoted as nutrient guidelines that meet the needs of most healthy individuals. Although these are adequate to prevent outright nutritional deficiency diseases such as scurvy, beriberi, and pellagra, they are not designed for optimal health. The Health LifeLine illustrated below runs the gamut from death at one end to optimal health and wellness at the other. The RDAs are sufficient to prevent most people from getting these severe nutritional deficiency diseases, which fall on the Health Line about where you see the X.

Death——**X**——————————————————————— **Optimal Health**
HEALTH LIFELINE

Does it make sense to consume just enough nutrients to keep you slightly beyond the X point on the Health LifeLine? Some health professionals refer to the RDAs as the "minimum wage of nutrition." We must recognize that RDAs don't address optimal health and wellness. In most cases, nutrient intakes necessary for optimal health are greater than the RDAs. We should not be satisfied with minimal health. We should aim for optimal health.

THE SAFETY OF NUTRITIONAL SUPPLEMENTS

Hundreds, perhaps thousands, of studies have reported that doses of nutrients higher than the RDAs provide significant health benefits. But it typically has taken decades for the research to filter down through health professionals to the general public.

A good example is the work of Dr. Kilmer McCully, who began publishing studies in 1969 showing that elevated blood homocysteine is a major risk factor for cardiovascular disease. At the time, tremendous amounts of research dollars and large professional egos were committed to the "cholesterol hypothesis." It has taken more than 30 years for Dr. McCully's message to receive widespread attention. Now we now know that additional levels of folic acid, vitamin B_6, and vitamin B_{12} will lower elevated homocysteine levels. Taking three B vitamins at levels above the RDA (costing only pennies per day) may be one of the most effective ways to decrease your risk of cardiovascular disease.

The issue of safety usually comes up when nutritional supplement recommendations above the RDA are suggested. The margin of error with most nutrients, however, is much broader than it is with prescription drugs. A case in point is a study titled "Incidence of Adverse Drug Reactions in Hospitalized Patients."[4] The authors of this study reported that in 1994 an estimated 2,216,000 hospitalized patients experienced a serious adverse drug reaction and in the same year an estimated 106,000 hospitalized patients died, not from mistakes but, instead, from what was believed to be the correct use of those medications. If outpatient drug-related deaths were considered, the figure undoubtedly would be much higher. This study implies that deaths related to the correct use of medications may rank among the leading causes of death in the United States.

Statistics compiled from the American Association of Poison Control Centers over an 8-year period also make a powerful statement. These statistics recorded the number of deaths reported at Poison Control Centers from prescription drugs, non-prescription drugs, and nutrients from 1987 through 1994.[5] During this period, there were 4,065 deaths from all drugs (prescription and non-prescription), compared to five deaths from nutrients, one of which was later determined to have been an error.

These studies suggest that drugs represent a much greater risk than nutritional supplements. The improper use of nutrients, however, can also cause problems. As examples, vitamin D and iron are two nutrients that can cause health problems if they are consumed in excessive quantities over time. Vitamin A and vitamin E, which are fat-soluble, and the trace mineral selenium are examples of nutrients that can produce toxic effects when they are taken in excess. Still, individuals would have to be grossly negligent over an extended time to create a problem with these nutrients. In general, the diseases developed, money lost, and the pain, suffering, and death that occur in individuals who do not ingest sufficient levels of nutrients for optimal health are much more significant than the occasional incident of toxic overdose of a nutrient.

In her book *New Passages*, Gail Sheehy notes that the aging process for health-conscious baby boomers is quite different than it was for previous generations.[6] Our parents made plans for retirement or actually retired between ages 55 and 65. Ms. Sheehy states that, at this age, health-conscious baby boomers can consider themselves "in the infancy of their second adulthood." A healthy extension of both quantity and quality of life is available to everyone.

The judicious use of nutritional supplements along with a healthy diet and lifestyle enable most individuals to have a great deal of control over their immune system and aging process. These are choices and decisions that every person can make for himself or herself that will have enormous impact on health, quality of life, and longevity. As Albert Szent–Gyorgy, discoverer of vitamin C, stated: "Active supplements are the least expensive, most effective health insurance you can buy."

For many people, the term "nutritional supplement" means vitamins. In reality, a lack of minerals is equally, if not more, problematic than a deficiency of vitamins. This is because most huge factory-farming organizations use chemical fertilizers that do not include trace minerals. Thus, the commercial food supply is experiencing a continual decline in the trace minerals that are essential nutrients. This is why individuals should take nutritional supplements containing a wide range of both vitamins and minerals.

Nutritional supplement programs vary considerably. Many nutritional supplements are one-tablet-daily formulations that contain RDA levels of nutrients, but the dosage recommendation for many high-potency nutritional supplements entails taking several tablets daily. These products have a twofold benefit:

1. They contain greater than RDA levels of nutrients, and taking them twice daily provides the additional benefit of maintaining a more even blood level of nutrients throughout the day

2. This, in turn, may increase antioxidant protection and help to slow the aging process.

In an article published in the June 19, 2002, issue of the *Journal of the American Medical Association* (*JAMA*), the respected physicians/ authors stated that a review of the scientific literature led them to recommend that all adults should take nutritional supplements. This represents a dramatic paradigm shift from the antinutritional-supplement stance that the medical professional has promoted and maintained for the past half century.

Greater stress, more environmental pollutants, poorer nutritional content of much of the food we eat, and the widespread use of medications that deplete nutrients — all point to the need today to take well-formulated, high-potency multivitamin/mineral supplements. At the very least, it is essential to consider taking the nutrients known to be depleted by medications we are taking. Although various companies provide nutrition-specific formulas for classes of drugs that deplete nutrients, we suggest that you check their formulas against the information in this book to assure proper nutrient replacement.

Our goal is to provide health education products and services that will enable and empower millions of Americans to have healthier, happier, longer lives. We hope this book helps you along this path.

NOTES

1. 38th Annual Survey of Top 200 Drugs, by IMS Health, *Pharmacy Times*, April 2002.
2. See Note 1.
3. Pot-Shot #1409, by A. Brilliant, Brilliant Enterprises, Santa Barbara, CA.
4. "Incidence of Adverse Drug Reactions in Hospitalized Patients: A Meta-analysis of Prospective Studies," by J. Lazarou, et al., *Journal of the American Medical Association*, Vol. 179, No. 15 (April 15, 1998), pp. 1200–1205.
5. Information supplied by Donald Loomis. Original data from the American Association of Poison Control Centers. Statistics first published in the *American Journal of Emergency Medicine*.
6. *New Passages* by Gail Sheehy (New York: Random House, 1995).

Part I *presents a synopsis of the drug classifications,*

the nutrient losses they can produce in the body,

and some of the potential health problems that can result.

Part II *expands upon this information,*

explaining what these drugs are

and expanding upon the health problems

and symptoms that can result from their use.

Quick Reference Guide to
NUTRITIONAL LOSSES

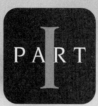

PART I

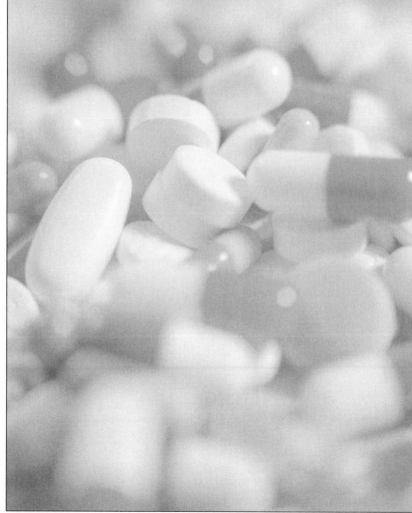

Drug	Nutrient Losses	Some Potential Health Problems
ANTACIDS		
■ MAGNESIUM & ALUMINUM ANTACIDS	*Calcium* *Phosphorus* *Folic acid*	Osteoporosis, heart & blood pressure problems, tooth decay Skeletal problems, anxiety, nervousness Anemia, birth defects, cervical dysplasia, heart disease, cancer risk
■ SODIUM BICARBONATE (Alka-Seltzer®, baking soda)	*Potassium* *Folic acid*	Irregular heartbeat, muscle weakness, fatigue, edema Anemia, birth defects, cervical dysplasia, heart disease, cancer risk
ANTI-ANXIETY (ANXIOLYTIC) DRUGS: BENZODIAZEPINES		
■ ALPRAZOLAM & DIAZEPAM	*Melatonin*	Insomnia/poor sleep, increased risk for breast cancer, reduced antioxidant status.
■ DIAZEPAM (Valium®), ALPRAZOLAM (Xanax®)	*Melatonin*	Insomnia, increased risk for cancer, increased free radical damage, which accelerates aging
ANTIBIOTICS		
■ GENERAL	*B vitamins* *Vitamin K* *Lactobacillus bifadus* *Bifidobacter bifidus*	Short-term depletion effects are minimal, but failure to reinoculate the GI tract with probiotics often results in dysbiosis, which causes gas & bloating and decreases the digestion & absorption of nutrients, and also may lead to a variety of other health problems. Diarrhea, increase in allergies, bloating, gas, epigastric pain and other digestive problems, malabsorption of vitamins/minerals, candida, other digestive problems. Everyone, from infants to the elderly, are urged to take probiotics (containing acidophilus & bifidus) twice daily during and after meals for 2 weeks after finishing a course of antibiotics.

Drug	Nutrients Depleted	Effects
■ AMINOGLYCOSIDES (amikacin, gentamicin, kanamycin, neomycin, streptomycin, tobramycin)	*B vitamins* *Beta-carotene* *Calcium* *Fat* *Iron* *Magnesium* *Nitrogen* *Potassium* *Sodium* *Vitamin A* *Vitamin K*	Minimal problems with short-term use
■ ANTI-MALARIAL	*Calcium* *Vitamin D*	Osteoporosis, heart & blood pressure problems, tooth decay Osteoporosis, muscle weakness, hearing loss
■ PENICILLINS	*Potassium*	Irregular heartbeat, muscle weakness, fatigue, edema
■ TETRACYCLINES	*Calcium* *Iron* *Magnesium* *Vitamin B$_6$* *Zinc*	Osteoporosis, heart & blood pressure irregularities, tooth decay Anemia, slow wound-healing, fatigue Cardiovascular problems, asthma, osteoporosis, muscular weakness & cramps, PMS, anxiety, nervousness, insomnia Depression, sleep disturbance, increased risk for cardiovascular disease Weak immunity, slow wound-healing, loss of senses of & taste, sexual dysfunction
■ TUBERCULOSIS-TREATING DRUGS cycloserine	*Calcium* *Folic acid*	Osteoporosis, heart & blood pressure problems, tooth decay Birth defects, cervical dysplasia, anemia, heart disease, cancer risk, depression

Drug	Nutrient Losses	Some Potential Health Problems
ANTIBIOTICS (Contd.)		
	Magnesium	Cardiovascular problems, palpitation, asthma, osteoporosis, muscular weakness & cramps, PMS, anxiety, nervousness
	Vitamin B$_3$	Skin, gastrointestinal, & nervous system problems
	Vitamin B$_6$	Depression, insomnia, cardiovascular risk
	Vitamin K	Anemia, depression, cardiovascular risk
ethambutol	*Copper*	Anemia, fatigue, cardiovascular & connective tissue problems
	Zinc	Weak immunity, slow wound-healing, loss of senses of smell & taste, sexual dysfunction
isoniazid (INH)	*Calcium*	Osteoporosis, heart & blood pressure problems, tooth decay, nervousness
	Vitamin B$_3$	Skin conditions, gastrointestinal & nervous system problems
	Vitamin B$_6$	Depression, insomnia, cardiovascular risk
	Vitamin D	Osteoporosis, muscle weakness, hearing loss
para-aminosalicylic acid	*Vitamin B$_{12}$*	Anemia, depression, cardiovascular problems
rifampin	*Vitamin D*	Osteoporosis, muscle weakness, hearing loss
■ TRIMETHOPRIM (Bactrim®, Proloprim® Septra®, Trimpex®)	*Folic acid*	Minimal problems with short-term use
ANTICONVULSANTS		
■ CARBAMAZEPINE (Tegretol®)	*Biotin* *DHA fatty acid*	Hair loss, depression, cardiac irregularities, dermatitis Skin problems (eczema, psoriasis), weight gain, memory problems, allergies, inflammatory problems (arthritis), blood sugar regulatory problems

Drug	Nutrient	Effects of Depletion
	Folic acid	Anemia, birth defects, heart disease, cervical dysplasia, cancer risk, depression
	Vitamin D	Osteoporosis, muscle weakness, hearing loss
	Vitamin E	Heart disease risk, weakened immune system, increased free radical damage
■ PHENOBARBITAL & BARBITURATES	*Calcium*	Osteoporosis, heart & blood pressure irregularities, tooth decay
	Folic acid	Anemia, birth defects, heart disease cervical dysplasia & cancer risk, depression
	Vitamin D	Osteoporosis, muscle weakness, hearing loss
	Vitamin K	Blood coagulation & skeletal problems
	Biotin	Hair loss, depression, cardiac irregularities, dermatitis
■ PHENYTOIN (Dilantin®)	*Biotin*	Hair loss, depression, cardiac irregularities, dermatitis
	Calcium	Osteoporosis, heart & blood pressure irregularities, tooth decay
	DHA fatty acid	Skin problems (eczema, psoriasis), weight gain, memory problems, allergies, inflammatory problems (arthritis), blood sugar regulatory problems
	Folic acid	Anemia, birth defects, cervical dysplasia, heart disease, cancer risk, depression
	Vitamin B$_1$	Depression, irritability, memory loss, muscle weakness, edema
	Vitamin B$_{12}$	Anemia, tiredness, weakness, increased risk for cardiovascular disease, neuropathy, depression
	Vitamin D	Osteoporosis, muscle weakness, hearing loss
	Vitamin E	Heart disease risk, weakened immune system, increased free radical damage
	Vitamin K	Blood coagulation & skeletal problems

Drug	Nutrient Losses	Some Potential Health Problems
ANTICONVULSANTS (Contd.)		
■ PRIMIDONE (Mysoline®)	*Biotin*	Hair loss, depression, cardiac irregularities, dermatitis
	DHA (fatty acid)	Skin problems (eczema, psoriasis), weight gain, memory problems, allergies, inflammatory problems (arthritis), blood sugar regulatory problems
	Folic acid	Anemia, birth defects, cervical dysplasia, heart disease, cancer risk, depression
■ VALPROIC ACID (Depakane®, Depakote®, Depacon®)	*Carnitine*	Muscle weakness & cramps, fatigue
	Copper	Anemia, fatigue, cardiovascular & connective tissue problems
	DHA (fatty acid)	Skin problems (eczema, psoriasis), weight gain, memory problems, allergies, inflammatory problems (arthritis), blood sugar regulatory problems
	Folic acid	Anemia, birth defects, cervical dysplasia, heart disease, cancer risk, depression
	Selenium	Lower immunity, reduced antioxidant protection
	Vitamin B6	Depression, sleep disturbance, increased risk for cardiovascular disease
	Vitamin E	Cardiovascular risk; cancers, PMS, macular degeneration
	Zinc	Weak immunity, slow wound-healing, loss of sense of smell & taste, sexual dysfunction
ANTIDIABETIC DRUGS		
■ BIGUANIDES metformin (Glucophage®)	*Vitamin B12*	Anemia, tiredness, weakness, increased risk for cardiovascular disease, depression

Drug	Nutrient Depleted	Potential Effects
	Coenzyme Q₁₀	Various cardiovascular problems, weakened immune system, low energy, muscle weakness, blood sugar regulation
	Folic acid	Anemia, birth defects, cervical dysplasia, heart disease, cancer risk, depression
■ SULFONYLUREAS acetohexamine (Dymelor®) glyburide (Micronase®/Glynase®/Dia Beta®) tolazamide (Tolinase®)	*Coenzyme Q₁₀*	Various cardiovascular problems, weakened immune system, low energy, muscle weakness, blood sugar regulation

ANTIFUNGAL DRUGS

Drug	Nutrient Depleted	Potential Effects
■ AMPHOTERICIN B	*Calcium* *Magnesium*	Osteoporosis, heart & blood pressure irregularities, tooth decay Cardiovascular problems, asthma, osteoporosis, PMS, nervousness, anxiety, insomnia, muscle weakness & cramps
	Potassium *Sodium*	Irregular heartbeat, muscle weakness, fatigue, edema Muscle weakness, memory loss, dehydration

ANTIHISTAMINES

Drug	Nutrient Depleted	Potential Effects
■ HYDROXYZINE (Atarax®, Vistaril®, & others)	*Melatonin*	Insomnia, increased risk for cancer, increased free radical damage contributing to aging

Drug	Nutrient Losses	Some Potential Health Problems
ANTI-INFLAMMATORY DRUGS		
■ CORTICOSTEROIDS prednisone methylprednisolone (Medrol®) triamcinolone (Aristocort®) dexamethasone (Decadron®)	*Calcium* *Chromium* *Folic acid* *Magnesium* *Potassium* *Selenium* *Vitamin B$_6$* *Vitamin B$_{12}$* *Vitamin C* *Vitamin D*	Osteoporosis, heart & blood pressure irregularities, tooth decay Elevated blood sugar, cholesterol & triglycerides, risk for diabetes Anemia, birth defects, cervical dysplasia, cardiovascular disease, depression Cardiovascular problems, palpitation, asthma, osteoporosis, PMS, anxiety, nervousness, insomnia, muscle weakness Irregular heartbeat, muscle weakness, fatigue, edema Lowered immunity, reduced antioxidant protection, increased risks for cardiovascular disease and cancer Depression, sleep disturbance, increased risk for cardiovascular disease Anemia, tiredness, weakness, increased risk for cardiovascular disease Lowered immunity, easy bruising, poor wound-healing Osteoporosis, muscle weakness, hearing loss
■ ASPIRIN & SALICYLATES	*Vitamin C* *Calcium* *Folic acid* *Iron* *Potassium* *Sodium* *Vitamin B$_5$*	Lowered immunity, easy bruising, poor wound-healing Osteoporosis, heart & blood pressure irregularities, tooth decay Anemia, birth defects, cervical dysplasia, cardiovascular disease, depression Anemia, weakness, fatigue, hair loss, brittle nails Irregular heartbeat, muscle weakness, fatigue, edema Muscle weakness, memory loss, dehydration Fatigue, listlessness, possible problems with skin, liver, & nerves

Drug	Nutrient	Effects
SULFASALAZINE (Azulfidine®)	*Folic acid*	Anemia, birth defects, cervical dysplasia, cardiovascular disease, depression
INDOMETHACIN (Indocin®)	*Folic acid*	Anemia, birth defects, cervical dysplasia, cardiovascular disease, depression
	Iron	Anemia, weakness, fatigue, hair loss, brittle nails
OTHER NSAIDS ibuprofen (Motrin®) sulindac (Clinoril®) mefenamic acid (Ponstel®) piroxicam (Feldene®) salsalate (Disalcid®) naproxen (Naprosyn®) & others	*Folic acid*	Anemia, birth defects, cervical dysplasia, cardiovascular disease, depression

ANTI-PARKINSON'S DISEASE DRUGS

Drug	Nutrient	Effects
LEVODOPA	*Potassium*	Irregular heartbeat, muscle weakness, fatigue, edema
	SAMe	Important for synthesis of many compounds & detoxification reactions
	Vitamin B$_6$	Depression, sleep disturbance, increased risk for cardiovascular disease

ANTI-PROTOZOAL DRUGS

Drug	Nutrient	Effects
PENTAMIDINE	*Magnesium*	Cardiovascular problems, palpitation, asthma, osteoporosis, PMS, anxiety, nervousness, insomnia, muscle weakness & cramps

Drug	Nutrient Losses	Some Potential Health Problems
ANTIVIRAL DRUGS		
■ FOSCARNET	*Calcium*	Osteoporosis, heart & blood pressure irregularities, tooth decay
	Magnesium	Cardiovascular problems, palpitation asthma, osteoporosis, PMS, nervousness, anxiety, muscle weakness & cramps, insomnia
	Potassium	Irregular heartbeat, muscle weakness, fatigue, edema
■ ZIDOVUDINE (Retrovir®, AZT, & other related drugs)	*Carnitine*	Increased blood lipids, abnormal liver function & glucose control
	Copper	Anemia, fatigue, cardiovascular & connective tissue problems
	Vitamin B$_{12}$	Anemia, tiredness, weakness, increased risk for cardiovascular disease
	Zinc	Weakened immunity, slow wound-healing, loss of senses of smell & taste, sexual dysfunction

BRONCHODILATORS

■ THEOPHYLLINE-CONTAINING DRUGS	*Vitamin B₆*	Depression, sleep disturbance, increased risk for cardiovascular disease
■ BETA₂ ADRENERGIC AGONISTS albuterol (Airet®, Proventil®, Ventolin®, Volmax®)	*Potassium*	Irregular heartbeat, muscle weakness, fatigue, edema
■ TERBUTALINE (Brethaire®, Brethine®, Bricanyl®)	*Potassium*	Irregular heartbeat, muscle weakness, fatigue, edema

CANCER CHEMOTHERAPY

	Many nutrients	Damage to the cells lining the GI tract, disruption of beneficial intestinal bacteria, nausea & vomiting, loss of appetite & inhibition of detoxification mechanisms, which can lead to multiple nutrient depletions.

Drug	Nutrient Losses	Some Potential Health Problems
CARDIOVASCULAR DRUGS		
■ ACE INHIBITORS	*Sodium*	Weak depletion; sodium supplementation or replacement is not warranted unless advised by a physician
captopril (Capoten®) enalapril (Vasotec®)	*Zinc*	Documented only in captopril & enalapril: lower immunity; slow wound-healing; loss of senses of smell & taste, sexual dysfunction
fosinopril (Monopril®) lisinopril (Prinovil®) quinapril (Accupril®) ramipril (Altace®) trandolapril (Mavik®)		
■ BETA-BLOCKERS propranolol (Inderal®) sotolol (Betapace®) nadolol (Corgard®) atenolol (Tenormin®) acebutolol (Sectral®) metoprolol (Lopressor®, Toprol®) timolol (Blocadren®) pindolol (Visken®) & others	*Coenzyme Q_{10}* *Melatonin*	Various cardiovascular problems, weakened immune system, low energy, muscle weakness, blood sugar regulation Insomnia, increased risk for breast cancer, increased free radical damage, aging acceleration

Drug Class	Nutrient Depleted	Symptoms
■ CALCIUM CHANNEL BLOCKERS nifedipine (Adalat®, Procardia®, & Procardia XL®) verapamil (Calan®, Covera®-HS, Isoptin®, Verelan®) nicardene (Cardene®) diltiazem (Cardizem®, Dilacor®, Tiazac®) felodipine (Plendil®) amlodipine (Norvasc®), & others	*Potassium*	Irregular heartbeat, muscle weakness, fatigue, edema
■ CARDIAC GLYCOSIDES digoxin (Lanoxin®)	*Calcium* *Magnesium* *Phosphorus* *Vitamin B$_1$*	Osteoporosis, heart & blood pressure irregularities, tooth decay Cardiovascular problems, palpitation, asthma, osteoporosis, PMS, anxiety, nervousness, muscle weakness & cramps, insomnia Weakness, low energy, skeletal problems Depression, irritability, memory loss, muscle weakness, edema
■ CENTRALLY ACTING ANTIHYPERTENSIVES clonidine (Catapres®) methyldopa (Aldomet®)	*Coenzyme Q$_{10}$*	Various cardiovascular problems, weakened immune system, low energy, muscle weakness, blood sugar regulation

Drug	Nutrient Losses	Some Potential Health Problems
CARDIOVASCULAR DRUGS (Contd.)		
■ HYDRALAZINE-CONTAINING VASODILATORS	*Vitamin B₆* *Coenzyme Q₁₀*	Depression, insomnia, risk for cardiovascular disease Various cardiovascular problems, weakened immune system, low energy, muscle weakness, blood sugar regulation
■ LOOP DIURETICS furosemide (Lasix®) bumetanide (Bumex®) ethacrynic acid (Edecrin®)	*Calcium* *Magnesium* *Potassium* *Vitamin B₁* *Vitamin B₆* *Vitamin C* *Sodium* *Zinc*	Osteoporosis, heart & blood pressure irregularities, tooth decay Cardiovascular problems, palpitation, asthma attacks, osteoporosis, PMS, anxiety, nervousness, insomnia, muscle weakness & cramps Irregular heartbeat, muscle weakness, fatigue, edema Depression, irritability, memory loss, muscle weakness, edema Depression, sleep disturbance, increased risk for cardiovascular disease Lowered immunity, easy bruising, poor wound-healing Muscle weakness, dehydration, memory problems, loss of appetite Weakened immunity, slow wound-healing, loss of senses of smell & taste, sexual dysfunction
■ POTASSIUM-SPARING DIURETICS Dyazide®, Maxzide®, Triamterene (Dyrenium®)	*Calcium* *Folic acid* *Zinc*	Osteoporosis, heart & blood pressure irregularities, tooth decay Anemia, birth defects, cervical dysplasia, cardiovascular disease, depression Weakened immunity, slow wound-healing, loss of senses of smell & taste, sexual dysfunction
■ THIAZIDE DIURETICS chlorothiazide (Diuril®) chlorthalidone (Hygroton®) hydrochlorothiazide (HCTZ) indapamide (Lozol®) metolazone (Zaroxolyn®), & others	*Coenzyme Q₁₀* *Magnesium* *Potassium* *Sodium* *Zinc*	Various cardiovascular problems, weakened immune system, low energy, muscle weakness, blood sugar regulation Cardiovascular problems, palpitation, asthma, osteoporosis, muscle weakness & cramps, PMS, anxiety, nervousness, insomnia Irregular heartbeat, muscle weakness, fatigue, edema Muscle weakness, dehydration, memory problems, loss of appetite Weakened immunity, slow wound-healing, loss of senses of smell & taste, sexual dysfunction

CHOLESTEROL-LOWERING DRUGS

■ BILE ACID
SEQUESTRANTS
cholestyramine
(Questran®)
colestipol
(Colestid®)

Beta-carotene
Calcium
Fat
Folic acid
Iron
Magnesium
Phosphorus
Vitamins A, D, E, K, B$_{12}$
Zinc

See Nutrient Reviews, Part III page 66

■ HMG-CoA REDUCTASE
INHIBITORS
atorvastatin (Lipitor®)
cerivastatin (Baycol®)
fluvastatin (Lescol®)
lovostatin (Advicor®,
  Mevacor®)
rosuvastatin calcium
  (Crestor®)
pravastatin (Pravacol®)
simvastatin (Zocor®)

Coenzyme Q$_{10}$

Various cardiovascular problems, weakened immunity, low energy, muscle weakness, blood sugar regulation

Drug	Nutrient Losses	Some Potential Health Problems
CHOLESTEROL-LOWERING DRUGS (Contd.)		
■ "FIBRATES" clofibrate (Atromid-S®) fenofibrate (TriCor®)	*Vitamin E*	Heart disease risk, weakened immune system, increased free radical damage
	Vitamin B$_{12}$	Anemia, tiredness, weakness, increased risk for cardiovascular disease, depression, neuropathy
	Copper	Anemia, fatigue, elevated cholesterol, connective tissue problems
	Zinc	Weakened immunity, slow wound-healing, loss of senses of smell & taste, sexual dysfunction
■ GEMFIBROZIL (Lopid®)	*Coenzyme Q$_{10}$*	Various cardiovascular problems, weakened immune system, low energy, muscle weakness, blood sugar regulation
	Vitamin E	Heart disease risk, weakened immune system, increased free radical damage
ELECTROLYTE REPLACEMENT		
■ POTASSIUM CHLORIDE (timed-release) (Micro-K® , Slow-K®)	*Vitamin B$_{12}$*	Anemia, tiredness, weakness, increased risk for cardiovascular disease, neurological complaints, depression

■ ORAL CONTRACEPTIVES (Estrogen replacement, ERT or Hormone replacement, HRT)	Calcium	Osteoporosis, heart & blood pressure irregularities, tooth decay
	Folic acid	Birth defects, cervical dysplasia, anemia, cardiovascular disease, depression, neuropathy,
	Tyrosine	lowered thyroid function
	Vitamin B_1	Depression, irritability, memory loss, muscle weakness, edema
	Vitamin B_2	Problems with skin, eyes, mucous membranes & nerves
	Vitamin B_3	Cracked, scaly skin, swollen tongue, diarrhea
	Vitamin B_6	Depression, sleep disturbances, increased risk for cardiovascular disease
	Vitamin B_{12}	Anemia, tiredness, weakness, increased risk for cardiovascular disease, depression, neuropathy
	Vitamin C	Lowered immunity, easy bruising, poor wound healing
	Vitamin E	High cholesterol, risk for cardiovascular diseases, cancers, PMS, macular degeneration
	Magnesium	Cardiovascular problems, asthma, osteoporosis, muscle cramps, PMS
	Selenium	Lowered immunity, reduced antioxidant protection, cardiovascular problems
	Tyrosine	thyroid and nuerotansmitter problems
	Zinc	Weak immunity, wound healing, senses of smell & taste, & sexual dysfunction

Drug	Nutrient Losses	Some Potential Health Problems
GOUT MEDICATIONS		
■ COLCHICINE (Col-benemid®)	*Beta-carotene*	Lowered immunity, reduced antioxidant protection
	Calcium	Osteoporosis, heart & blood pressure irregularities, tooth decay
	Phosphorus	Anxiety, skeletal problems
	Potassium	Irregular heartbeat, muscle weakness, fatigue, edema, nervous disorders
	Sodium	Muscle weakness, dehydration, loss of appetite, poor concentration
	Vitamin B$_{12}$	Anemia, tiredness, weakness, increased risk for cardiovascular disease, depression
LAXATIVES		
■ MINERAL OIL Agoral®, Haley's M-O®	*Beta-carotene,* *Vitamin A, D, E, K, &* *beta-carotene*	Multiple problems associated with depletion of fat-soluble nutrients
	Calcium	Osteoporosis, heart & blood pressure irregularities, tooth decay
	Phosphorus	Anxiety, skeletal problems
■ BISACODYL Bisac-Evac®, Bisacodyl Uniserts®, Bisco-Lax® Carter's Little Pills® Clysodrast®, Dacodyl® Deficol®, Dulcolax® Feen-A-Mint®, Fleet® Laxative	*Potassium*	Irregular heartbeat, muscle weakness, fatigue, edema

Drug	Nutrient	Effects
■ PHOSPHATE ENEMA Fleet® enema	*Calcium* *Magnesium*	Osteoporosis, heart & blood pressure irregularities, tooth decay Cardiovascular problems, palpitation, asthma, osteoporosis, muscle weakness & cramps, PMS, anxiety, nervousness, insomnia

PSYCHOTHERAPEUTIC DRUGS

Drug	Nutrient	Effects
■ TRICYCLIC ANTIDEPRESSANTS amitriptyline (Elavil®) desipramine (Norpramin®) nortriptyline (Aventyl®, Pamelor®) doxepin (Sinequan®) imipramine (Tofranil®) & others	*Coenzyme Q_{10}* *Vitamin B_2*	Various cardiovascular problems, weakened immunity, low energy, muscle weakness, blood sugar regulation Problems with skin, eyes, mucous membranes, & nerves
■ PHENOTHIAZINES chlorpromazine (Thorazine®) thioridazine (Mellaril®) fluphenazine (Permitil®, Prolixin®) mesoridazine (Serentil®) & others	*Coenzyme Q_{10}* *Vitamin B_2* *Melatonin*	Various cardiovascular problems, weakened immunity, low energy, muscle weakness, blood sugar regulation Problems with skin, eyes, mucous membranes, & nerves Insomnia, increased cancer risk, increased aging from free radical damage

Drug	Nutrient Losses	Some Potential Health Problems
PSYCHOTHERAPEUTIC DRUGS (Contd.)		
■ MONOAMINE OXIDASE INHIBITORS (MAOs) phenelzine (Nardil®)	*Vitamin B$_6$*	Depression, sleep disturbance, increased risk for cardiovascular disease
■ BUTYROPHENONES haloperidol (Haldol®)	*Melatonin* *Vitamin E*	Insomnia, increased cancer risk, increased aging from free radical damage Depression, sleep disturbance, increased risk for cardiovascular disease
■ LITHIUM Eskalith®, Lithobid®, Lithonate®, Lithotabs®	*Inositol*	Excessive urination & excessive thirst
■ SSRIs (selective serotonin reuptake inhibitors) Celexa®, Luvox®, Paxil®, Prozac®, Zoloft®	*Sodium*	Weakness, fatigue, cardiovascular problems, nausea, vomiting, bloating, cramping
STEROIDS, ANABOLIC		
■ STANOZOLOL (Winstrol®)	*Iron*	Anemia, weakness, fatigue, hair loss, brittle nails

■ LEVOTHYROXINE (Levothroid®, Levoxyl®, Synthroid®, & others)	*Iron*	Anemia, weakness, fatigue, hair loss, brittle nails

ULCER MEDICATIONS

■ H-2 BLOCKERS cimetidine (Tagamet®) famotidine (Pepcid®) nizatidine (Axid®) ranitidine (Zantac®)	*Vitamin B$_{12}$*	Anemia, tiredness, weakness, increased risk for cardiovascular disease, depression, neuropathy
	Calcium	Osteoporosis, heart & blood pressure irregularities, tooth decay
	Folic acid	Anemia, birth defects, cervical dysplasia, cardiovascular disease, depression, cancer risk
	Iron	Anemia, weakness, fatigue, hair loss, brittle nails
	Protein	Potential amino acid deficiencies
	Vitamin D	Osteoporosis, muscle weakness, hearing loss
	Zinc	Weak immunity, slow wound-healing, loss of senses of smell & taste, sexual dysfunction
■ PROTON PUMP INHIBITORS lansoprazole (Prevacid®) omeprazole (Prilosec®) pantoprazole (Protonix®) rabeprazole (Aciphex®) esomeprazole (Nexium®)	*Vitamin B$_{12}$*	Anemia, tiredness, weakness, increased risk for cardiovascular disease, depression
	Protein	Potential amino acid deficiencies

Drug	Nutrient Losses	Some Potential Health Problems
MISCELLANEOUS		
■ EDTA	*Calcium*	Osteoporosis, heart & blood pressure irregularities, tooth decay
■ METHOTREXATE	*Folic acid*	Birth defects, cervical dysplasia, anemia, cardiovascular disease, depression
■ PENICILLAMINE	*Copper*	Anemia, fatigue, elevated cholesterol, connective tissue problems
	Magnesium	Cardiovascular problems, palpitation, asthma, osteoporosis, PMS, anxiety, nervousness, muscle weakness & cramps, insomnia
	Vitamin B_6	Depression, sleep disturbance, increased risk for cardiovascular disease
	Zinc	Weak immunity, wound healing, loss of senses of smell & taste, sexual dysfunction
■ RITODRINE	*Calcium*	Osteoporosis, heart & blood pressure irregularities, tooth decay
	Potassium	Irregular heartbeat, muscle weakness, fatigue, edema

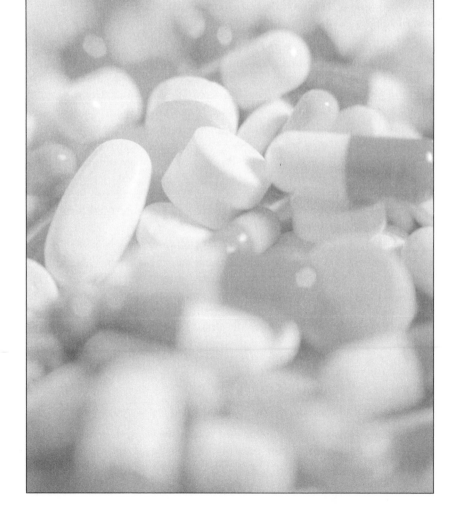

NUTRITION

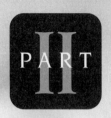

PART
II

ANTACIDS

Antacids are of two primary types — those containing magnesium and aluminum salts and those that contain sodium bicarbonate.

■ MAGNESIUM/ALUMINUM HYDROXIDE ANTACIDS

Antacids containing magnesium/aluminum hydroxide deplete calcium, phosphate, and folic acid.

Many over-the-counter antacids contain a combination of magnesium and aluminum salts. The aluminum in these products can bind with phosphate in the intestinal tract, preventing absorption and resulting in lower levels of phosphate in the blood. To compensate for this loss, the body begins to release both phosphate and calcium from skeletal stores in the bones. Excess calcium eventually is lost through the urine. The gastrointestinal tract also becomes less acidic, which inhibits the absorption of folic acid.

• *Antacids containing magnesium/aluminum hydroxide and calcium depletion:* Insufficient calcium can result in skeletal problems such as osteoporosis and osteomalacia. Calcium deficiency also can cause high blood pressure, muscle cramps, heart palpitation, tooth decay, back and leg pains, insomnia, and nervous disorders.

• *Antacids containing magnesium/aluminum hydroxide and phosphate depletion:* A deficiency in phosphate can result in skeletal problems, as well as anxiety or nervousness. People who use magnesium/aluminum antacids only occasionally are not likely to be affected by these problems. Nevertheless, many people (especially the elderly) use these products regularly to alleviate symptoms of gastrointestinal distress, and frequent use can lead to problems.

• *Antacids containing magnesium/aluminum hydroxide and folic acid depletion:* A deficiency of folic acid can cause anemia, birth defects, cervical dysplasia, elevated homocysteine level, headache, fatigue, depression, hair loss, anorexia, insomnia, diarrhea, nausea, and increased susceptibility to infections. Folic acid deficiency also is associated with greater risk for developing breast cancer and colorectal cancer. For a more detailed description of folic acid deficiency problems, see Female Hormones, pages 69–75.

■ SODIUM BICARBONATE ANTACIDS

Antacids containing sodium bicarbonate deplete potassium and folic acid.

• *Sodium bicarbonate antacids and potassium depletion:* Short-term or occasional use of sodium bicarbonate antacids is not likely to cause health problems. Many people (especially the elderly), however, use these products regularly to alleviate the symptoms of indigestion. Frequent use of sodium bicarbonate antacids can cause potassium depletion. Symptoms associated with potassium depletion include irregular heartbeat, poor reflexes, muscle weakness, fatigue, continuous thirst, edema, constipation, dizziness, mental confusion, and nervous disorders.

• *Sodium bicarbonate antacids and folic acid depletion:* Folic acid deficiency can cause anemia, birth defects, cervical dysplasia, elevated homocysteine, headache, fatigue, depression, hair loss, anorexia, insomnia, diarrhea, nausea, and increased infections. Folic acid deficiency also is associated with increased risk for developing breast cancer and colorectal cancer. For a more detailed description of folic acid deficiency problems, see pages 110–113.

ANTI-ANXIETY AGENTS: BENZODIAZEPINES

In 2002, the drug class benzodiazepines, which represents the primary class of anti-anxiety medications, had four individual drugs in the top 200 drugs of the year in terms of sales. Benzodiazepines, as a class, are the best-selling drugs in the history of medicine, with annual worldwide sales of $21 billion.[1]

■ DIAZEPAM AND ALPRAZOLAM

The benzodiazepines diazepam and alprazolam deplete melatonin.

Because melatonin is the brain hormone that triggers or induces sleep, a deficiency of melatonin results in insomnia and related sleep problems. Insomnia can lead to many other problems, including depression, poor performance at work, and an increase in accidents. Insufficiency of melatonin also hinders the release of growth hormone, causes changes in blood sugar, and may promote inflammation chemistry.

Melatonin is also an important antioxidant, so a depletion of melatonin could result in more damage to free radicals and an acceleration of the aging process. Finally, numerous studies have associated low levels of melatonin with an increased incidence of breast cancer.

ANTIBIOTICS

Virtually all antibiotics affect the overall health of the gastrointestinal tract. If the beneficial bacteria in the intestinal tract are not replaced following a course of antibiotics, a condition known as dysbiosis can develop, and this can cause additional nutrient depletion. The use of antibiotics also depletes the B vitamins and vitamin K. The discussion of antibiotics here refers to the effects of the following classes of antibiotics: penicillins, cephalosporins, fluoroquinolones, macrolides, aminoglycosides, and sulfonamides.

Advances in technology over the past several decades have produced quantum leaps in our understanding of the many important health benefits of the "friendly bacteria" in the human intestinal tract. Scientists have discovered that intestinal bacteria are intimately involved in functions such as digesting and absorbing nutrients, producing vitamins, preventing various forms of cancer, detoxifying pollutants, and metabolizing cholesterol. The beneficial bacteria also provide resistance to infections and control and influence our immune system.

The use of antibiotics has grown enormously over the last few decades. During the 1990s, doctors in the United States wrote from 200 to 250 million prescriptions for antibiotics each year. In 2002, U.S. sales of the drug class that contains antibiotics (called anti-infective agents) ranked fifth in all the drug classes, with total sales of more than $24 billion annually.[2]

Although the discovery and use of antibiotics has boosted the health and longevity of people in the 20th century, this widespread use has had some serious health consequences. One of the main problems associated with the use of antibiotics is that they disrupt the normal balance of bacteria in the intestinal tract. Unfortunately, antibiotics kill the beneficial bacteria along with the pathological species. If an individual does not reinoculate the intestinal tract with beneficial bacteria, or probiotics, other organisms have the opportunity to grow and proliferate. This can result in a variety of health problems, both mental and physical. Disruption of the normal microflora in the intestinal tract causes a health problem termed dysbiosis.

Once a person has received a prescription for antibiotics, he or she should take large doses of probiotics twice daily with meals while on the antibiotic medicine and for one week after discontinuing the medication. The person should take the probiotics 2 hours apart. This helps to rebuild and restore the population of friendly bacteria in the intestinal tract. The most common of the beneficial bacteria are *Lactobacillus acidophilus* (or *L. acidophilus*) and *bifidobacteria bifidum* (or bifidus).

The use of antibiotics can cause nutrient depletions through three different mechanisms:

1. The friendly bacteria normally manufacture a wide variety of vitamins in the intestinal tract. Antibiotics kill off the beneficial bacteria, and this effectively stops the production of these vitamins, which include vitamin B_1 (thiamin), vitamin B_2 (riboflavin), vitamin B_3 (niacin), vitamin B_5 (pantothenic acid), vitamin B_6 (pyridoxine), vitamin B_{12} (cobalamin), biotin, inositol, and vitamin K.

2. The friendly bacteria produce a wide range of enzymes that aid in the digestion and absorption of nutrients. When antibiotics kill off the beneficial bacteria, digestion suffers and fewer nutrients are absorbed.

3. If probiotics are not consumed following a course of antibiotics, unfavorable organisms are likely to grow, and this can create additional health problems For example, candida yeast organisms can proliferate and secrete toxins into the body.

Scientists have not yet been able to design studies that determine the precise nutritional effects of the vitamins that the beneficial bacteria in our bodies produce. Still, numerous studies and clinical observations indicate that many people develop significant health problems arising from an imbalance of the bacterial flora in the gastrointestinal tract following the use of antibiotics.

Bacterial imbalance in the intestinal tract can cause a wide range of symptoms and problems throughout the body. Frequently, a person has symptoms in a part of the body far removed from the intestines and therefore does not realize that the problem stems from toxins produced by unfavorable bacteria in the intestinal tract. Symptoms or disorders that can be caused by dysbiosis include acne, diarrhea, constipation, PMS, hormonal problems, easy bruising, candida yeast infections, chronic vaginal and bladder infections, food allergies, bad breath, osteoporosis, anemia, anxiety, B-vitamin deficiency, general malabsorption, and nutrient depletion.

The beneficial intestinal bacteria also manufacture vitamin K, a nutrient that regulates blood-clotting mechanisms and calcium deposition into the bone matrix. Thus, a deficiency of vitamin K can cause coagulation problems, which in turn can result in bleeding and hemorrhage. Vitamin K deficiency also may be associated with skeletal problems such as osteoporosis.

■ ANTIBIOTICS TO TREAT TUBERCULOSIS

The antibiotics used to treat tuberculosis are isoniazid, ethambutol, rifampin, cycloserine, and para-aminosalicylic acid.

Isoniazid

Isoniazid has been reported to deplete vitamin B_3, vitamin B_6, vitamin D, and calcium.

• *Isoniazid and niacin depletion:* Vitamin B_3 (niacin) depletion can produce skin, intestinal, and nervous system problems. These conditions usually develop only with a critical deficiency of niacin.

• *Isoniazid and vitamin B_6 depletion:* Vitamin B_6 (pyridoxine) depletion can cause depression, insomnia, and increased risk for cardiovascular disease.

– *Depression:* Vitamin B_6 is necessary to convert the amino acid tryptophan into the neurotransmitter serotonin. A deficiency of serotonin in the brain is strongly associated with depression. Therefore, people taking drugs that deplete vitamin B_6 are at greater risk for developing depression.

– *Insomnia:* In the brain, serotonin is converted into melatonin, a hormone that controls sleep. Because a vitamin B$_6$ deficiency inhibits the synthesis of serotonin, it also will decrease the amount of melatonin that can be produced in the brain. People who become deficient in melatonin are likely to have insomnia and related sleep problems.

– *Cardiovascular disease:* Vitamin B$_6$ is one of the B vitamins necessary to metabolize homocysteine, an amino acid produced from the metabolism of the essential amino acid methionine. Homocysteine is a toxic substance capable of directly injuring the lining of the arteries — the type of damage that causes atherosclerosis. Under normal conditions, homocysteine exists only briefly. A lack of vitamin B$_6$, however, produces elevated levels of homocysteine in the blood. Even slight elevations of homocysteine represent a seriously increased risk for developing atherosclerosis, the leading cause of heart disease.

• *Isoniazid and vitamin D depletion:* Vitamin D depletion can lead to osteoporosis and other skeletal problems. Because vitamin D is necessary for calcium absorption, a vitamin D deficiency could cause a calcium deficiency as well. Vitamin D depletion also can result in muscle weakness and hearing loss.

• *Isoniazid and calcium depletion:* Vitamin D is necessary for calcium absorption. With the depletion of vitamin D, calcium could be depleted along with it. This can lead to osteoporosis, heart irregularities, elevated blood pressure, and tooth decay.

Ethambutol

Ethambutol has been reported to deplete zinc and copper.

• *Ethambutol and zinc depletion:* Zinc is a mineral important to the immune system. Its deficiency can weaken the immune system and result in slow healing of wounds. Zinc deficiency also causes loss of the senses of taste and smell and can produce infertility and sexual dysfunction in men and women.

• *Ethambutol and copper depletion:* Insufficient copper can result in anemia and fatigue, problems with maintenance and repair of connective tissues, and elevated serum cholesterol.

Rifampin

Rifampin has been reported to deplete vitamin D.

• Vitamin D is necessary for calcium absorption, which means that a vitamin D deficiency could produce a calcium deficiency. Vitamin D depletion, therefore, can result in osteoporosis and other skeletal problems. Vitamin D depletion also can cause muscle weakness and hearing loss.

Cycloserine

Cycloserine has been reported to deplete vitamin B_3, vitamin B_6, vitamin B_{12}, calcium, magnesium, vitamin K, and folic acid.

• **Cycloserine and vitamin B_3 depletion:** Vitamin B_3 (niacin) depletion can produce problems with the skin, intestinal, and nervous systems. These problems usually develop only with a critical deficiency of niacin.

• **Cycloserine and vitamin B_6 depletion:** Vitamin B_6 (pyridoxine) depletion can cause depression, insomnia, and increased risk for cardiovascular disease.

• **Cycloserine and vitamin B_{12} depletion:** A vitamin B_{12} deficiency can cause anemia, accompanied by fatigue, tiredness, and weakness. A B_{12} deficiency also is a common contributor to depression, especially in the elderly population. Inadequate levels of B_{12} result in an elevated homocysteine level, which poses a greatly increased risk for cardiovascular disease. If serious B_{12} deficiencies are not corrected, they can lead to long-term, irreversible neurological damage.

• **Cycloserine and calcium depletion:** Vitamin D is necessary for calcium absorption. Because cycloserine causes a depletion of vitamin D, calcium could be depleted, too. This can lead to osteoporosis, heart irregularities, elevated blood pressure, and tooth decay.

• **Cycloserine and magnesium depletion:** Magnesium depletion can cause cardiac arrhythmias, high blood pressure, and various other cardiovascular-related problems. Additional conditions associated with low magnesium levels are osteoporosis, muscle cramps and muscular weakness, fatigue, anxiety, nervousness, insomnia, PMS, and an increase in the frequency and severity of asthma attacks.

• **Cycloserine and vitamin K depletion:** Because vitamin K regulates blood-clotting mechanisms, a deficiency of vitamin K can cause problems with coagulation. This, in turn, can result in bleeding and hemorrhage. Newborn babies have a higher risk of hemorrhaging problems if the mother has been taking vitamin K-depleting antibiotic drugs such as cycloserine. Vitamin K also is necessary for bone metabolism, and its deficiency may contribute to bone loss.

• **Cycloserine and folic acid depletion:** Depletion of folic acid can produce some serious health problems, especially in women. Folic acid deficiency disrupts DNA metabolism, which leads to the production of abnormal cells. This problem is especially acute in cells with the most rapid rates of turnover, including red blood cells, white blood cells, leukocytes, and epithelial cells of the stomach, intestine, vagina, and uterine cervix.

Folic acid needs are greater during pregnancy. Folic acid insufficiency also is one of the most common vitamin deficiencies. In addition to people not eating enough green leafy vegetables, folic acid is easily destroyed by heat, light, and oxygen, and substantial losses occur during food processing, cooking, and storage.

Folic acid deficiency can cause anemia, birth defects, cervical dysplasia, elevated homocysteine levels, headache, fatigue, depression, hair loss, anorexia, insomnia, diarrhea, nausea, and increased infections. Further, folic acid deficiency is associated with increased risk for developing breast cancer and colorectal cancer.

The following is a synopsis of the major health problems related to deficiency of folic acid. These problems affect women more than men and point out the need for supplementation in many circumstances.

- *Anemia:* Folic acid is required for the production of red blood cells (erythrocytes), which carry oxygen from the lungs to the tissues and carbon dioxide from the tissues to the lungs. Folic acid deficiency results in reduced tissue oxygenation. This causes a condition known as megaloblastic anemia, with symptoms of tiredness, weakness, diarrhea, and weight loss.

- *Birth defects:* Folic acid helps regulate neural (nerve) development and the transfer of genetic material to new cells in the fetus. During pregnancy, the rapidly growing fetus substantially increases a woman's need for folic acid, and folic acid deficiency during pregnancy dramatically increases the risk for birth defects including spina bifida and cleft palate. The link between folic acid deficiency and birth defects is so strong that all women of childbearing age are urged to have their folic acid status checked before trying to become pregnant. If this practice were followed, thousands of birth defects probably would be prevented each year. A laboratory test called the Neutrophilic Hypersegmentation Index (NHI) easily identifies folic acid insufficiency.

- *Cervical dysplasia:* The development of abnormal cells in the uterus, cervical dysplasia is regarded as a precancerous condition that usually is discovered when a woman has a Pap exam. This condition could contribute to an increased number of hysterectomies. Approximately 800,000 women have hysterectomies every year in the United States. Some health-care professionals believe that the folic acid depletion attributed to taking oral contraceptives and other medications is linked to this high incidence of cervical dysplasia and hysterectomies.

– *Elevated homocysteine,* also known as hyperhomocysteinemia, now is recognized as a serious independent risk factor for cardiovascular disease. Excess homocysteine is capable of directly damaging the vascular endothelial cells, causing the type of damage that initiates plaque build-up in the arteries. Even moderate elevations of homocysteine represent substantially increased risk for plaque build-up and blood clots.

Para-aminosalicylic Acid

Para-aminosalicylic acid has been reported to deplete Vitamin B_{12}:

• *Para-aminosalicylic acid and vitamin B_{12} depletion:* A vitamin B_{12} deficiency can cause anemia, accompanied by fatigue, tiredness, and weakness. A B_{12} deficiency also is a common contributor to depression, especially in the elderly population. Inadequate levels of B_{12} result in an elevated homocysteine level, which poses a greatly increased risk for cardiovascular disease. If serious B_{12} deficiencies are not corrected, they can lead to long-term, irreversible neurological damage.

■ AMINOGYLCOSIDES

Aminogylcosides are broad-spectrum antibiotics that are used both topically (on the skin) and internally. Drugs that belong to the aminoglycoside class of antibiotics include amikacin, gentamicin, kanamycin, neomycin, streptomycin, and tobramycin. Topical application for short periods of time is of minimal concern. When amnioglycosides are taken internally, however, they can deplete many nutrients including calcium, magnesium, nitrogen, potassium, sodium, vitamin, A, beta-carotene, fat, and the full range of B vitamins and vitamin K that the beneficial bacteria in the intestinal tract normally produce.

Rather than discuss each of these potential nutrient depletions separately, individuals using any of these drugs are encouraged to consult each of the nutritional reviews in Part III and the introduction to Antibiotics, pages 27–35. These discussions emphasize the importance of replenishing the beneficial bacteria in the gastrointestinal tract.

■ ANTIMALARIAL ANTIBIOTICS

Antimalarial antibiotics deplete hydroxychloroquine.

• *Hydroxychloroquine and calcium and vitamin D depletion:* Hydroxyquinone given to a patient undergoing long-term dialysis leads to a decrease in calcium and vitamin D. After discontinuation of the drug, levels of Vitamin D and calcium return to normal. Long-term therapy with the antimalarial drug hydroxchloroquine may result in osteoporosis, osteopenia, and other skeletal diseases.

■ PENICILLIN ANTIBIOTICS

Penicillin antibiotics deplete potassium.

• **Penicillin antibiotics and potassium depletion:** Many of the various types of penicillin antibiotics have been reported to deplete potassium. Potassium depletion can produce muscular weakness, tetany (muscle spasms), and postural hypotension (low blood pressure when changing from a lying or sitting position to a standing position), which in turn can cause dizziness and fainting spells. Other symptoms associated with potassium depletion are irregular heartbeat, poor reflexes, fatigue, continuous thirst, edema, constipation, mental confusion, and nervous disorders. In a hospital setting, symptoms usually are treated and managed by giving intravenous potassium chloride.

■ TETRACYCLINE ANTIBIOTICS

Short-term use of tetracycline antibiotics — 1 to 2 weeks to treat an infection — is not likely to cause a significant depletion of nutrients. Nevertheless, if probiotics are not taken during and after the course of antibiotics to reestablish the population of beneficial bacteria in the intestinal tract, a number of health problems can develop (see pages 27–29).

One of the biggest problems associated with tetracyclines use arises when doctors prescribe them for teenage acne. In these cases, children are directed to take doses of the antibiotic daily, often for years. This can seriously disrupt the intestinal microflora, causing dysbiosis, which can result in nutritional depletions and other health problems. Therefore, probiotics should be used daily, even with low-dose antibiotic therapy. Tetracycline antibiotics easily react with and prevent the absorption of minerals including calcium, iron, magnesium, and zinc.

Tetracycline antibiotics deplete calcium, magnesium, iron, and zinc, as well as the full range of B vitamins and vitamin K that the beneficial bacteria in the intestinal tract normally produce. (See the introduction to Antibiotics, pages 27–29.

• **Tetracyclines and calcium depletion:** Calcium depletion leads to skeletal problems such as osteoporosis (porous, brittle bones that break easily) and osteomalacia (gradual softening and bending of the bones with varying severity of pain). Calcium deficiency also can cause high blood pressure, heart palpitation, muscle cramps, tooth decay, back and leg pains, insomnia, and nervous disorders.

• **Tetracyclines and iron depletion:** Iron depletion causes anemia and the accompanying weakness and fatigue. Iron depletion also causes slow healing of wounds and general weakening of the immune system. Nevertheless, iron supplementation is not recommended unless a lab test determines that iron deficiency is present.

- **Tetracyclines and magnesium depletion:** Magnesium depletion can cause cardiac arrhythmias, high blood pressure, and various other cardiovascular-related problems. Additional conditions associated with low magnesium levels are osteoporosis, muscle cramps, PMS, and an increase in the frequency and severity of asthma attacks.

- **Tetracyclines and zinc depletion:** The mineral zinc is important to a healthy immune system. A deficiency of zinc can cause slow healing of wounds and a weakened immune system, as well as a loss of the senses of taste and smell. Zinc deficiency also can result in infertility and sexual dysfunction in men and women.

■ TRIMETHOPRIM

Trimethoprim causes the depletion of folic acid.

Antibiotics containing trimethoprim cause a minor depletion of folic acid. As with antibiotics in general, killing off beneficial bacteria in the intestines reduces the production of all the B vitamins and vitamin K. Because these antibiotics usually are taken for only a short period of time, these depletions probably are insignificant. Nevertheless, if probiotics are not taken during and after the course of antibiotics to reestablish the population of beneficial bacteria in the intestinal tract, a number of health problems can develop (see pages 27–29).

ANTICONVULSANTS

In 1998, the most current year for the statistics on anticonvulsants (also referred to as anti-seizure medications), this category of prescription drugs ranked 10th in dollar-volume in the United States, accounting for more than $2 billion in sales. In terms of numbers of prescriptions, this class of drugs was 17th in 1998, with 43,918,000 prescriptions written.[3]

Each of the anticonvulsant drugs — barbiturates, phenytoin, carbamazepine, primidone, and valproic acid — will be discussed separately, along with the nutrients they deplete. All anticonvulsants deplete folic acid.

■ BARBITURATES

Barbiturates can cause the depletion of calcium, folic acid, vitamin D, vitamin K, and biotin.

- **Barbiturates and calcium depletion:** Barbiturates and most of the other anticonvulsant drugs cause a decrease in the intestinal absorption of calcium, which results in increased fecal excretion of calcium. Thus, individuals taking these medications are at increased risk for developing a calcium deficiency. Calcium supplementation will not solve this problem because the calcium deficiency is the result of a vitamin D deficiency and vitamin D is necessary for calcium absorption. Barbiturates inhibit vitamin D production in the body, and this in turn decreases calcium absorption. To solve the problem, individuals should be given vitamin D supplements to facilitate normalization of calcium absorption.

Calcium depletion can result in skeletal problems such as rickets in children and osteomalacia or osteoporosis in adults. Rickets and osteomalacia are essentially the same condition, characterized by gradual softening and bending of the bones with varying severity of pain. Osteoporosis is characterized by porous, brittle bones that break easily. Calcium deficiency also can cause high blood pressure, muscle cramps, heart palpitation, tooth decay, back and leg pains, insomnia, and nervous disorders.

• *Barbiturates and folic acid depletion:* Folic acid deficiency can lead to some serious health problems, especially in women. Folic acid deficiency disrupts DNA metabolism, which causes the production of abnormal cells. This problem is especially acute in cells with the most rapid turnover rates — red blood cells, white blood cells, and epithelial cells of the stomach, intestine, vagina, and uterine cervix. The need for folic acid is greater during pregnancy.

Insufficient folic acid is one of the most common vitamin deficiencies. In addition to people not eating enough green leafy vegetables, folic acid is easily destroyed by heat, light, and oxygen. Substantial losses also occur during food processing, cooking, and storage. Folic acid deficiency can cause anemia, birth defects, cervical dysplasia, elevated homocysteine, headache, fatigue, depression, hair loss, anorexia, insomnia, diarrhea, nausea, and increased infections. Folic acid deficiency also is associated with increased risk for developing breast cancer and colorectal cancer.

The major health issues related to folic acid deficiency are reviewed below. These health problems underscore the importance of individuals (especially women) taking folic acid supplementation.

– *Anemia:* Folic acid is required for the production of erythrocytes (red blood cells), which carry oxygen from the lungs to the tissues and carbon dioxide from the tissues to the lungs. Folic acid deficiency produces anemia and reduced tissue oxygenation, which in turn leads to a condition known as megaloblastic anemia, with symptoms including tiredness, weakness, diarrhea, and weight loss.

– *Birth defects:* Folic acid helps regulate neural development in the fetus, and the transfer of genetic material to new cells. During pregnancy, the rapidly growing fetus substantially increases a woman's need for folic acid, and folic acid deficiency during pregnancy dramatically increases the risk for birth defects such as spina bifida and cleft palate. The link between folic acid deficiency and birth defects is so strong that all women of childbearing age are urged to have their folic acid status checked before trying to become pregnant. If this practice were followed, thousands of birth defects probably would be prevented each year. A laboratory test, the Neutrophilic Hypersegmentation Index (NHI), easily identifies folic acid insufficiency.

– *Cervical dysplasia*: The development of abnormal cells in the uterus, cervical dysplasia, is a precancerous condition. It usually is discovered when a woman has her Pap exam. This condition may contribute to the number of hysterectomies — approximately 800,000 every year in the United States. Some health-care professionals believe that the folic acid depletion caused by oral contraceptives and other medications is linked to this high incidence of cervical dysplasia and hysterectomies.

– *Elevated homocysteine*: Also known as hyperhomocysteinemia, a high level of homocysteine is now recognized as a serious independent risk factor for cardiovascular disease. Excess homocysteine can cause direct damage to vascular endothelial cells, the type of damage that initiates plaque build-up in the arteries. Even moderate elevation of homocysteine represents substantially increased risk for plaque build-up and blood clots.

Note. Physicians are urged to use caution when administering megadose folic acid therapy to patients who are on anticonvulsant medications, as there is a report of intravenous folic acid administration inducing a seizure in one patient.

• *Barbiturates and vitamin D depletion:* Vitamin D depletion can lead to rickets in children and osteomalacia and osteoporosis in adults. These skeletal problems develop because vitamin D is necessary for calcium absorption. Vitamin D deficiency conditions result from insufficient deposition of calcium phosphate into the bone matrix. In children, this produces bones that are not strong enough to withstand the ordinary stresses and strains of weight-bearing, which can result in muscle weakness, pain, knock-knees, bowed legs, spinal curvature, pigeon breast, disfiguring of the skull, and tooth decay and dental problems. Lack of vitamin D in adults causes osteoporosis, a condition in which the bones become thin, porous, and more likely to fracture. Vitamin D deficiency also can result in hearing loss.

• *Barbiturates and vitamin K depletion:* Because vitamin K regulates blood-clotting mechanisms, a deficiency of vitamin K can produce coagulation problems, which can result in bleeding and hemorrhage.

The trauma of birthing can cause life-threatening intracranial bleeding in infants born to mothers who have been taking the barbiturate phenobarbital during pregnancy. Vitamin K also is necessary for bone metabolism, and its insufficiency may contribute to bone loss.

• *Barbiturates and biotin depletion:* Biotin deficiency can result in hair loss, depression, skin problems, and elevated blood glucose and cholesterol levels.

■ PHENYTOIN

Patients who are prescribed phenytoin usually have to take the drug for the rest of their lives. This long-term use can cause many health problems directly related to the nutritional depletions that the drug causes.

The most serious of the problems caused by depletion of these nutrients are birth defects as a result of folic acid deficiency in pregnant women and skeletal problems in children and adults alike from vitamin D and calcium depletions. Vitamin B_1 deficiency resulting from phenytoin therapy also has been reported to lower IQ scores. Two other potential problems are increased rates of depression and cardiovascular disease as a result of folic acid and vitamin B_{12} depletion.

Phenytoin can cause the depletion of a wide range of nutrients including biotin, calcium, folic acid, vitamin B_1, vitamin B_{12}, vitamin D, vitamin E, DHA fatty acid, and vitamin K.

• *Phenytoin and biotin depletion:* Biotin deficiency can result in hair loss, depression, skin problems, and elevated blood glucose and cholesterol levels.

• *Phenytoin and calcium depletion:* Insufficiency of phenytoin and most of the other anticonvulsant drugs causes a decrease in the intestinal absorption of calcium, which results in increased fecal excretion of calcium. Therefore, individuals taking these medications are at increased risk for developing a calcium deficiency. Calcium supplementation is not an appropriate way to solve this problem because the calcium deficiency is actually the result of a vitamin D deficiency and vitamin D is necessary for calcium absorption. Barbiturates inhibit vitamin D production in the body, and this in turn decreases calcium absorption. To solve the problem, patients have to be given vitamin D supplements, which facilitate normalization of calcium absorption.

Calcium depletion can result in skeletal problems such as rickets in children and osteoporosis or osteomalacia in adults. These diseases are characterized by gradual softening and bending of the bones with varying severity of pain. Calcium deficiency also can cause high blood pressure, muscle cramps, heart palpitation, tooth decay, back and leg pains, insomnia, and nervous disorders.

• *Phenytoin and folic acid depletion:* All anticonvulsant drugs deplete folic acid. This depletion can cause some serious health problems, especially in women, and folic acid needs are greater during pregnancy.

Folic acid deficiency disrupts DNA metabolism, which results in the production of abnormal cells. This problem is especially acute in cells with the most rapid rates of turnover, including red blood cells, white blood cells, epithelial cells of the stomach, intestine, vagina, and uterine cervix.

Deficiency of folic acid is one of the most common vitamin deficiencies. In addition to people not eating enough green leafy vegetables, folic acid is easily destroyed by heat, light, and oxygen, and substantial losses occur during food processing, cooking, and storage.

Folic acid deficiency can cause anemia, birth defects, cervical dysplasia, elevated homocysteine levels, headache, fatigue, depression, hair loss, anorexia, insomnia, diarrhea, nausea, and increased infections. Folic acid deficiency is associated with higher risk for developing breast cancer and colorectal cancer. The following is a synopsis of the major health problems related to folic acid deficiency. These conditions affect women more than men and point up the need for supplementation in many circumstances.

– *Anemia:* Folic acid is required for the production of erythrocytes (red blood cells), which carry oxygen from the lungs to the tissues and carbon dioxide from tissues to the lungs. Folic acid deficiency results in reduced tissue oxygenation. This causes a condition known as megaloblastic anemia, with symptoms of tiredness, weakness, diarrhea, and weight loss.

– *Birth defects:* Folic acid helps regulate neural development and the transfer of genetic material to new cells in the fetus. During pregnancy, the rapidly growing fetus substantially increases a woman's need for folic acid, and folic acid deficiency during pregnancy dramatically increases the risk for birth defects such as spina bifida and cleft palate. The link between folic acid deficiency and birth defects is so strong that all women of childbearing age are urged to have their folic acid status checked before trying to become pregnant. If this practice were followed, thousands of birth defects probably would be prevented each year. A laboratory test, the Neutrophilic Hypersegmentation Index (NHI), easily identifies folic acid insufficiency.

– *Cervical dysplasia:* The development of abnormal cells in the uterus, cervical dysplasia, is regarded as a precancerous condition that usually is discovered when a woman has a Pap exam. This condition could contribute to an increased number of hysterectomies.

Approximately 800,000 women have hysterectomies every year in the United States. Some health care professionals believe that the folic acid depletion caused by oral contraceptives and other medications is linked to this high incidence of cervical dysplasia and hysterectomies.

 – *Elevated homocysteine,* also known as hyperhomocysteinemia, now is recognized as a serious independent risk factor for cardiovascular disease. Excess homocysteine is capable of directly damaging the vascular endothelial cells, causing the type of damage that initiates plaque build-up in the arteries. Even moderate elevations of homocysteine represent substantially increased risk for plaque build-up and blood clots.

Note. Physicians are urged to use caution when administering megadoses of folic acid therapy to patients who are taking anticonvulsant medications. One case has been reported of intravenous folic acid administration inducing a seizure.

• *Phenytoin and vitamin B_1 depletion:* A deficiency of vitamin B_1 can cause depression, irritability, memory loss, muscle weakness, and edema. One study noted that administration of vitamin B_1 with individuals who have a B_1 deficiency resulted in improvement in both verbal and nonverbal IQ scores.

• *Phenytoin and vitamin B_{12} depletion:* A vitamin B_{12} deficiency can cause anemia, which results in fatigue, tiredness, and weakness. A B_{12} deficiency also is a common cause of depression, especially in the elderly population. Inadequate levels of B_{12} result in elevated homocysteine, which poses a greatly increased risk for cardiovascular disease. If serious B_{12} deficiencies are not corrected, they can lead to long-term irreversible neurological damage.

• *Phenytoin and vitamin D depletion:* Vitamin D depletion can cause rickets in children and osteomalacia and osteoporosis in adults. These skeletal problems develop because vitamin D is necessary for calcium absorption. In children, vitamin D deficiency causes insufficient deposition of calcium phosphate into the bone matrix. This produces bones that are not strong enough to withstand the ordinary stresses and strains of weight-bearing and can result in muscle weakness, pain, knock-knees, bowed legs, spinal curvature, pigeon breast, disfiguring of the skull, and tooth decay and dental problems. When insufficient vitamin D results in a calcium deficiency in adults, it leads to osteoporosis, which makes the bones thin, porous, and more likely to fracture. Vitamin D deficiency also can result in hearing loss.

• *Phenytoin and vitamin E depletion:* Vitamin E is an important fat-soluble antioxidant. Vitamin E reduces the blood "stickiness" that may contribute to cardiovascular diseases such as atherosclerosis and high cholesterol levels. Vitamin E also helps to protect our bodies against cancers and other diseases such as PMS and macular degeneration.

• *Phenytoin and DHA depletion:* DHA is an essential omega-3 fatty acid that is an important component of brain and nerve tissue. Depletion of DHA can lead to various neurologic function problems as well as decline in memory.

• *Phenytoin and vitamin K depletion:* Because vitamin K regulates blood-clotting mechanisms, a deficiency of vitamin K can cause problems with coagulation. This, in turn, can result in bleeding and hemorrhage. Newborn babies have a higher risk of hemorrhaging problems if the mother has been taking vitamin K-depleting anticonvulsant drugs such as phenytoin. Vitamin K also is necessary for bone metabolism and its deficiency may contribute to bone loss.

■ CARBAMAZEPINE

Carbamazepine can deplete biotin, folic acid, DHA fatty acid, vitamin D, and vitamin E.

• *Carbamazepine and biotin depletion:* Biotin deficiency can result in hair loss, depression, skin problems, and an elevation of blood glucose and cholesterol levels.

• *Carbamazepine and folic acid depletion:* All anticonvulsant drugs deplete folic acid. This depletion can result in some serious health problems, especially in women, and folic acid needs are greater during pregnancy. Folic acid deficiency disrupts DNA metabolism, which causes abnormal cells to be produced. This problem is especially acute in cells with the most rapid rates of turnover, including red blood cells, leukocytes, and epithelial cells of the stomach, intestine, vagina, and uterine cervix.

Insufficient folic acid also is one of the most common vitamin deficiencies. In addition to people not eating enough green leafy vegetables, folic acid is easily destroyed by heat, light, and oxygen, and substantial losses occur during food processing, cooking, and storage.

Folic acid deficiency can cause anemia, birth defects, cervical dysplasia, elevated homocysteine, headache, fatigue, depression, hair loss, anorexia, insomnia, diarrhea, nausea, and increased infections. Folic acid deficiency also has been associated with increased risk of developing breast cancer and colorectal cancer. The following discussion goes into more detail about the major folic acid deficiency-related health problems. Folic acid supplementation, for women in particular, may be indicated.

- *Anemia:* Folic acid is required for the production of erythrocytes (red blood cells), which carry oxygen from the lungs to the tissues and carbon dioxide from the tissues to the lungs. Folic acid deficiency causes anemia and reduced tissue oxygenation. This results in a condition known as megaloblastic anemia, with symptoms of tiredness, weakness, diarrhea, and weight loss.

- *Birth defects:* Folic acid helps to regulate neural development in the fetus, as well as the transfer of genetic material to new cells. During pregnancy, the rapidly growing fetus substantially increases a woman's need for folic acid, and folic acid deficiency during pregnancy dramatically increases the risk of birth defects such as spina bifida and cleft palate. The link between folic acid deficiency and birth defects is so strong that all women of childbearing age are urged to have their folic acid status checked before trying to become pregnant. If this practice were followed, thousands of birth defects probably would be prevented each year. A laboratory test, the Neutrophilic Hypersegmentation Index (NHI), easily identifies folic acid insufficiency.

- *Cervical dysplasia:* The development of abnormal cells in the uterus, cervical dysplasia, is regarded as a precancerous condition that usually is discovered when a woman has her Pap exam. This condition might contribute to an increased number of hysterectomies. More than 800,000 women have hysterectomies every year in the United States, and some health-care professionals believe that the folic acid depletion caused by oral contraceptives and other medications is linked to this high incidence of cervical dysplasia and hysterectomies.

- *Elevated homocysteine:* Also known as hyperhomocysteinemia, elevated homocysteine is recognized as a serious independent risk factor for cardiovascular disease. Excess homocysteine can cause direct damage to vascular endothelial cells, leading to the conditions allowing plaque build-up in the arteries. Even moderate elevations of homocysteine represent substantially increased risk for the development of plaque build-up and blood clots.

Note. Physicians are urged to use caution when administering megadoses of folic acid to patients who are on anticonvulsant medications, as intravenous folic acid administration induced a seizure in one reported patient.

- *Carbamazepine and DHA depletion:* DHA is an omega-3 fatty acid that is an important component in brain and nerve tissue. Depletion of DHA can lead to various neurologic function problems and decline in memory.

• *Carbamazepine and vitamin D depletion:* Vitamin D depletion can cause rickets in children and osteomalacia and osteoporosis in adults. These skeletal problems develop because vitamin D is necessary for the absorption of calcium. In children, the vitamin D deficiency causes insufficient deposition of calcium phosphate into the bone matrix. This produces bones that are not strong enough to withstand the ordinary stresses and strains of weight bearing, which can result in muscle weakness, pain, knock-knees, bowed legs, spinal curvature, pigeon breast, a disfiguring of the skull, and tooth decay and dental problems. In adults, a lack of vitamin D causes a calcium deficiency, which leads to osteoporosis, in which the bones are thin, porous, and more likely to fracture. A vitamin D deficiency also can result in hearing loss.

• *Carbamazepine and vitamin E depletion:* Vitamin E is an important fat-soluble antioxidant. Vitamin E reduces the blood "stickiness" that contributes to cardiovascular diseases such as atherosclerosis and high cholesterol levels. Vitamin E also protects against cancers and other diseases such as PMS and macular degeneration.

■ PRIMIDONE

Primidone can cause the depletion of biotin and folic acid.

As with other anticonvulsant drugs, the most significant problems are to the skeletal system, arising from vitamin D and calcium depletion, as well as potential birth defects resulting form folic acid depletion in pregnant women.

• *Primidone and biotin depletion:* Biotin deficiency can result in hair loss, depression, skin problems, and an elevation of blood glucose and cholesterol levels.

• *Primidone and folic acid depletion:* All anticonvulsant drugs deplete folic acid. This depletion can incite some serious health problems, especially in women. Folic acid needs are greater during pregnancy. Folic acid deficiency disrupts DNA metabolism, which leads to the production of abnormal cells. This problem is especially acute in cells with the most rapid rates of turnover, including red blood cells, white blood cells, and epithelial cells of the stomach, intestine, vagina, and uterine cervix.

Folic acid deficiency is one of the most common vitamin deficiencies in the United States. In addition to people eating insufficient green leafy vegetables, folic acid is easily destroyed by heat, light, and oxygen. Food processing, cooking, and storage also destroy folic acid.

An insufficiency of folic acid can cause anemia, birth defects, cervical dysplasia, elevated homocysteine level, headache, fatigue, depression, hair loss, anorexia, insomnia, diarrhea, nausea, and increased infections. Folic acid deficiency also has been associated with increased risk for developing breast cancer and colorectal cancer. The major folic acid deficiency-related health problems are explored in more detail below. Folic acid supplementation may be advisable, particular for women.

- *Anemia:* Folic acid is required for the production of erythrocytes (red blood cells), which carry oxygen from the lungs to the tissues and carbon dioxide the tissues to the lungs. Folic acid deficiency results in anemia and reduced tissue oxygenation. The resulting condition, called megaloblastic anemia, produces symptoms of tiredness, weakness, diarrhea, and weight loss.

- *Birth defects:* Folic acid helps to regulate neural development and the transfer of genetic material to new cells. During pregnancy the rapidly growing fetus substantially increases the woman's need for folic acid, and folic acid deficiency during pregnancy dramatically increases the risk for birth defects such as spina bifida and cleft palate. The link between folic acid deficiency and birth defects is so strong that all women of childbearing age are advised to have their folic acid status checked before trying to become pregnant. If this practice were followed, thousands of birth defects probably would be prevented annually. A laboratory test, the Neutrophilic Hypersegmentation Index (NHI), is used to identify folic acid insufficiency.

- *Cervical dysplasia:* The development of abnormal cells in the uterus, cervical dysplasia is regarded as a precancerous condition. It usually is discovered at the time a woman has a Pap exam. This condition may contribute to an increased number of hysterectomies. (Approximately 800,000 women have hysterectomies every year in the United States.) Some health-care professionals believe that the folic acid depletion caused by oral contraceptives and other medications is linked to the high incidence of cervical dysplasia and hysterectomies.

- *Elevated homocysteine:* Also known as hyperhomocysteinemia, elevated homocysteine is recognized as an independent risk factor for cardiovascular disease. Because excessive homocysteine can cause direct damage to vascular endothelial cells, it can lead to plaque build-up in the arteries. Even moderate elevations of homocysteine represent substantially increased risk for plaque build-up and blood clots.

Note. Physicians are urged to use caution when administering megadoses of folic acid to patients who are taking anticonvulsant medications, following a report of seizure induced by intravenous folic acid administration.

■ VALPROIC ACID

Valproic acid can cause the depletion of folic acid, carnitine, copper, selenium, vitamin B_6, vitamin E, DHA fatty acid, and zinc.

• *Valproic acid and folic acid depletion:* A deficiency of folic acid can cause a wide range of health problems including anemia, depression, cervical dysplasia, birth defects, and increased risks for developing cardiovascular disease, breast cancer, and colorectal cancer. For a detailed discussion of the problems associated with folic acid deficiency, see the discussion of barbiturates and folic acid depletion, pages 35–38.

• *Valproic acid and carnitine depletion:* Carnitine is an amino acid that facilitates the transport of fats across cellular membranes for metabolism and the production of energy. Although the body normally makes adequate levels of carnitine, administration of valproic acid can create a carnitine deficiency, with symptoms of fatigue, muscle weakness, and muscular cramps.

• *Valproic acid and copper depletion:* Copper depletion can cause anemia and fatigue, problems with the maintenance and repair of connective tissues, and elevated levels of serum cholesterol.

• *Valproic acid and selenium depletion:* Selenium is an important antioxidant nutrient. A deficiency of selenium increases the risk for diseases such as cancer and cardiovascular disease. People who are selenium-deficient are subjected to increased free radical damage, which accelerates the aging process.

• *Valproic acid and vitamin E:* Vitamin E is an important fat-soluble antioxidant. Vitamin E reduces the blood "stickiness" that may contribute to cardiovascular diseases such as atherosclerosis and high cholesterol levels. Vitamin E also helps to protect the body against cancers and other diseases such as PMS and macular degeneration.

• *Valproic acid and DHA fatty acid depletion:* DHA is an omega-3 fatty acid that is an important component in brain and nerve tissue. Depletion of DHA can lead to various neurologic function problems and decline in memory.

• *Valproic acid and zinc depletion:* Zinc is an important mineral for a healthy immune system. Zinc deficiency can cause slow healing of wounds and a weakened immune system, as well as a loss of the senses of taste and smell. Zinc deficiency also can cause infertility and sexual dysfunction in men and women.

ANTIDIABETIC DRUGS

In 2000, oral antidiabetics—drugs used to treat non-insulin-dependent diabetes—were the tenth-largest therapeutic class, with a sales growth rate of 23% from 1996 to 2000. As a class, they increased in value from $2.4 billion in 1996 to $5.9 million in 2000. This represents 1.9% of global pharmaceutical sales. Bristol-Myers Squibb's Glucophage® dominated this class in 2000, with a market share of 31.5%, following sales growth of 33% over the year 2001.[4]

■ SULFONYLUREAS

Sulfonylureas deplete coenzyme Q_{10}.

• *Sulfonylureas and Q_{10} depletion:* Coenzyme Q_{10} is an extremely important antioxidant and also performs vital roles in generating energy in the mitochondria of all cells. The heart is the most active muscle in the human body, so a decline in energy resulting from a deficiency of CoQ_{10} first affects the heart, and now it is thought that a CoQ_{10} deficiency may be one of the primary causes of congestive heart failure.

In addition to providing antioxidant protection within the mitochondria, coenzyme Q_{10} protects LDL-cholesterol from free radical oxidation. Individuals who are deficient in coenzyme Q_{10} are at increased risk for cardiovascular disease and also have more free radical damage, which accelerates the aging process.

■ BIGUANIDES

Biguanides deplete vitamin B_{12}, coenzyme Q_{10}, and folic acid.

• *Biguanides and vitamin B_{12} depletion:* One study reported that 30% of individuals taking biguanides developed an inability to absorb vitamin B_{12}. In this study, 50% of individuals who developed biguanide-related vitamin B_{12} deficiency actually developed a permanent inability to produce intrinsic factor.[5] Because intrinsic factor is necessary for B_{12} absorption, these people may require vitamin B_{12} therapy indefinitely. Vitamin B_{12} depletion also can result in elevated levels of homocysteine, which poses a serious risk for cardiovascular disease. A long-term vitamin B_{12} deficiency can also result in irreversible nerve damage.

• *Biguanides and coenzyme Q_{10} depletion:* Coenzyme Q_{10} is an extremely important antioxidant and also performs vital roles in generating energy in the mitochondria of all cells. The heart is the most active muscle in the human body, so a decline in energy from a deficiency of CoQ_{10} first affects the heart, and now it is thought that a CoQ_{10} deficiency may be one of the primary causes of congestive heart failure. In addition to providing antioxidant protection within the mitochondria, CoQ_{10} protects LDL-cholesterol from free radical oxidation. Individuals who have a deficiency of CoQ_{10} are at increased risk for cardiovascular disease and also have more free radical damage, which accelerates the aging process.

• *Biguanides and folic acid depletion:* Folic acid depletion can cause some serious health problems, especially in women. Folic acid needs are greater during pregnancy. Folic acid deficiency disrupts DNA metabolism, which causes the production of abnormal cells. This problem is especially acute in cells with the most rapid rates of turnover, including red blood cells, white blood cells, and epithelial cells of the stomach, intestine, vagina, and uterine cervix. Insufficient folic acid is one of the most common vitamin deficiencies. In addition to people not eating enough green leafy vegetables, folic acid is easily destroyed by heat, light, and oxygen, as well as food processing, cooking, and storage.

Folic acid deficiency can cause anemia, birth defects, cervical dysplasia, elevated homocysteine, headache, fatigue, depression, hair loss, anorexia, insomnia, diarrhea, nausea, and increased infections. Folic acid deficiency also is associated with increased risk for breast cancer and colorectal cancer. The following list is a review the major folic acid deficiency-related health problems.

– *Anemia:* Folic acid is required for the production of erythrocytes (red blood cells), which carry oxygen from the lungs to the tissues and carbon dioxide from the tissues to the lungs. Folic acid deficiency results in anemia and reduced tissue oxygenation. This causes a condition called megaloblastic anemia, which produces symptoms of tiredness, weakness, diarrhea, and weight loss.

– *Birth defects:* Folic acid helps to regulate neural development and the transfer of genetic material to new cells in the fetus. During pregnancy, the rapidly growing fetus substantially increases a woman's need for folic acid, and folic acid deficiency during pregnancy dramatically increases the risk for birth defects such as spina bifida and cleft palate. The link between folic acid deficiency and birth defects is so strong that all women of childbearing age are advised to have their folic acid status checked before trying to become pregnant. If this practice were followed, thousands of birth defects probably would be prevented each year. A laboratory test, the Neutrophilic Hypersegmentation Index (NHI), easily identifies folic acid insufficiency.

– *Cervical dysplasia:* The development of abnormal cells in the uterus, cervical dysplasia, is regarded as a precancerous condition that usually is discovered when a woman has a Pap exam. This condition might contribute to an increased number of hysterectomies. Approximately 800,000 women have hysterectomies every year in the United States. Some health care professionals believe that the folic acid depletion caused by oral contraceptives and other medications is linked to the high incidence of cervical dysplasia and hysterectomies.

– *Elevated homocysteine,* also known as hyperhomocysteinemia, is recognized as an independent risk factor for cardiovascular disease. Excess homocysteine is capable of directly damaging vascular endothelial cells, causing the type of damage that initiates plaque build-up in the arteries. Even moderate elevation of homocysteine represents substantially increased risk for plaque build-up and blood clots.

ANTIFUNGALS: AMPHOTERICIN B

Antifungal medications have become more and more prevalent over the last decade. Although no nutrient depletions for oral antifungal medications are noted to date, it is an important category to foster the research as this category of drugs continues to escalate.

Amphotericin B depletes calcium, magnesium, potassium, and sodium.

Amphotericin B remains the antifungal drug of choice for most systemic infections. A limiting factor for its use is the development of kidney toxicity. Amphotericin B-induced kidney toxicity causes a build-up of nitrogen compounds in the blood, renal tubular acidosis, impaired renal concentrating ability, and electrolyte abnormalities including depletion of potassium, sodium, and magnesium. All of these abnormalities develop to varying degrees in almost all patients who receive the drug. Upon withdrawal of therapy, renal function gradually returns to baseline, although in some instances the person sustains permanent damage, especially when the cumulative dose exceeds 5g.

ANTIHISTAMINES: HYDROXYZINE

Of the many antihistamine medications, the only one on which studies on nutrient depletions have been conducted is hydroxyzine.

Hydroxyzine depletes melatonin.

Melatonin is the brain hormone that triggers or induces sleep. A deficiency of melatonin results in insomnia and related sleep problems. Insomnia can lead to many other problems such as depression, poor performance at work, and an increase in accidents. Melatonin also is an important antioxidant, so a depletion of melatonin could result in more free radical damage and acceleration of the aging process. Last, but not least, numerous studies have associated low levels of melatonin with an increased incidence of breast cancer.

ANTI-INFLAMMATORY DRUGS

In 2000, anti-inflammatory drugs, also called anti-arthritic medications, represented the 13th largest category of prescription drugs in the United States in terms of dollar volume, accounting for more than $9.5 billion in sales.

The categories of anti-inflammatory drugs are corticosteroids, salicylates (aspirin), sulfasalazine, indomethacin, and nonsteroidal anti-inflammatory drugs (NSAIDs). They are discussed below, along with the nutrients they deplete.

■ CORTICOSTEROIDS

Corticosteroids (glucocorticoids) can cause depletion of calcium, vitamin D, potassium, zinc, magnesium, vitamin C, folic acid, vitamin B$_{12}$, selenium, chromium, and vitamin A.

Corticosteroid-induced nutrient depletions are of minimal importance when the drugs are taken for only a short period, as is the case with dosepaks, which provide 21 tablets to be taken within 6 days. People who are on long-term therapy with corticosteroid drugs, however, can develop significant nutrient depletion-related health problems. Each of the nutrient depletions mentioned above are discussed individually along with their associated health problems.

• *Corticosteroids and calcium depletion:* Corticosteroids cause increased urinary excretion of calcium. The resulting calcium depletion increases the probability of developing skeletal problems such as rickets in children and osteoporosis and osteomalacia in adults. These problems can produce soft, weak bones, resulting in skeletal deformities. In adults, calcium-depleted bones are more likely to incur fractures. Calcium deficiency also can cause high blood pressure, muscle cramps, heart palpitation, tooth decay, back and leg pains, insomnia, and nervous disorders.

• *Corticosteroids and vitamin D depletion:* Treatment with corticosteroids does not directly deplete vitamin D but, by causing a depletion of calcium, creates a greater need for vitamin D to increase calcium absorption. Thus, by creating an indirect need for more vitamin D, corticosteroids can cause a vitamin D deficiency.

• *Corticosteroids and potassium depletion:* Corticosteroids cause increased urinary excretion of potassium, which can lead to hypokalemia (potassium depletion). This can be characterized by muscular weakness, tetany (muscle spasms), and postural hypotension (low blood pressure when changing from a lying or sitting position to a standing position), which can cause dizziness and fainting spells. Other symptoms associated with potassium depletion are irregular heartbeat, poor reflexes, fatigue, continuous thirst, edema, constipation, mental confusion, and nervous disorders.

• *Corticosteroids and zinc depletion:* The use of corticosteroids can weaken the immune system and cause slow-healing of wounds. Zinc deficiency also can result in insulin resistance, a loss of the senses of taste and smell, and infertility and sexual dysfunction in men and women alike.

• *Corticosteroids and magnesium depletion:* Corticosteroids cause increased urinary excretion of magnesium, which depletes magnesium levels in the body. Magnesium deficiency can produce cardiac arrhythmias, palpitation, high blood pressure, and various other cardiovascular-related problems, osteoporosis, muscle cramps and muscular weakness, PMS, anxiety, nervousness, insomnia, and an increase in the frequency and severity of asthma attacks.

• *Corticosteroids and vitamin C depletion:* The immune system can be weakened by the depletion of vitamin C resulting from use of corticosteroids. Low levels of vitamin C can accelerate aging damage because of increased free radical damage. In one study, ophthalmologists expressed their concern that vitamin C depletion might increase the risk for glaucoma and cataracts.

• *Corticosteroids and folic acid depletion:* Folic acid depletion can cause some serious health problems, especially in women, and folic acid needs are greater during pregnancy. Folic acid deficiency disrupts DNA metabolism, which results in the production of abnormal cells. This problem is especially acute in cells with the most rapid rates of turnover — red blood cells, white blood cells, and epithelial cells of the stomach, intestine, vagina, and uterine cervix. Insufficient folic acid also is one of the most common vitamin deficiencies. In addition to people not eating enough green leafy vegetables, folic acid is easily destroyed by heat, light, and oxygen, as well as food processing, cooking, and storage.

Folic acid deficiency can cause anemia, birth defects, cervical dysplasia, elevated homocysteine, headache, fatigue, depression, hair loss, anorexia, insomnia, diarrhea, nausea, and increased infections. Folic acid deficiency is associated with greater risk for developing breast cancer and colorectal cancer. The following paragraphs go into more detail about the major folic acid deficiency-related health problems, emphasizing the importance of individuals, especially women, receiving folic acid supplementation.

– *Anemia:* Folic acid is required for the production of erythrocytes, the red blood cells that carry oxygen from the lungs to the tissues and carbon dioxide from the tissues to the lungs. Folic acid deficiency results in anemia and reduced tissue oxygenation. This leads to a condition known as megaloblastic anemia, accompanied by symptoms of tiredness, weakness, diarrhea, and weight loss.

– *Birth defects:* Folic acid helps to regulate neural development and the transfer of genetic material to new cells in the fetus. During pregnancy, the rapidly growing fetus substantially increases a woman's need for folic acid, and folic acid deficiency during pregnancy dramatically increases the risk of birth defects such as spina bifida and cleft palate. The link between folic acid deficiency and birth defects is so strong that it is advisable for all women of childbearing age to have their folic acid status checked before trying to become pregnant. If this practice were followed, thousands of birth defects probably would be prevented each year. A laboratory test, the Neutrophilic Hypersegmentation Index (NHI), easily identifies folic acid insufficiency.

– *Cervical dysplasia:* The development of abnormal cells in the uterus, cervical dysplasia, is regarded as a precancerous condition that usually is discovered when a woman has a Pap exam. This condition can contribute to an increased number of hysterectomies. Approximately 800,000 women have hysterectomies every year in the United States. Some health-care professionals believe that the folic acid depletion caused by oral contraceptives and other medications is linked to the high incidence of cervical dysplasia and hysterectomies.

– *Elevated homocysteine:* Also known as hyperhomocysteinemia, elevated homocysteine is recognized as a serious independent risk factor for cardiovascular disease. Excess homocysteine can directly damage vascular endothelial cells. Therefore, it can cause the type of damage that initiates plaque build-up in the arteries. Even moderate elevations of homocysteine represent substantially increased risk for plaque build-up and blood clots.

• *Corticosteroids and vitamin B_{12} depletion:* A deficiency of vitamin B_{12} can cause anemia, characterized by tiredness, weakness, and fatigue. Inadequate vitamin B_{12} also can cause elevated levels of homocysteine, a risk factor for cardiovascular disease. Long-term B_{12} deficiency can result in permanent nerve damage. Another common manifestation of vitamin B_{12} deficiency is depression, especially in the elderly population.

• *Corticosteroids and selenium depletion:* Selenium is an important antioxidant nutrient, and its deficiency increases the risk for cancer and cardiovascular disease. People who are selenium-deficient are subjected to increased free radical damage, which accelerates the aging process.

• *Corticosteroids and chromium depletion:* Chromium deficiency can cause problems with blood sugar regulation, insulin resistance, and elevated cholesterol and triglycerides.

• *Corticosteroids and vitamin A depletion:* Insufficient vitamin A weakens the immune system and increases the risks for infections. This is because vitamin A is necessary for healthy mucous membranes, which are an important part of the immune system that functions as a barrier against infections. Vitamin A deficiency also can cause dry skin and problems with vision.

■ SALICYLATES (ASPIRIN)

Salicylates cause the depletion of vitamin C, calcium, folic acid, iron, sodium, potassium, and pantothenic acid (vitamin B$_5$).

• *Salicylates and vitamin C depletion:* Salicylates cause increased urinary excretion of vitamin C. In fact, the authors of one study stated that aspirin is the drug most likely to deplete vitamin C. Vitamin C deficiency can cause substantial weakening of the immune system and increased free radical damage, which accelerates the aging process.

• *Salicylates and calcium depletion:* Salicylates cause increased urinary excretion of calcium. Calcium depletion resulting from regular or long-term use increases the possibility of developing skeletal problems such as rickets in children and osteoporosis and osteomalacia in adults. These problems produce soft, weak bones, resulting in skeletal deformities. In adults, calcium-depleted bones are more likely to fracture. Calcium deficiency also can cause high blood pressure, muscle cramps, heart palpitation, tooth decay, back and leg pains, insomnia, and nervous disorders.

• *Salicylates and folic acid depletion:* Folic acid depletion can lead to a wide range of health problems including anemia, depression, and elevated homocysteine, which poses a seriously increased risk for cardiovascular disease. Folic acid deficiency also increases the risk for developing breast and colorectal cancers. The babies of women who become deficient in folic acid are at greater risk for birth defects, and their mothers for developing cervical dysplasia. (For a detailed discussion of folic acid deficiency problems, see pages 50–51.)

• *Salicylates and iron depletion:* Iron depletion can cause anemia, accompanied by weakness and fatigue. Other symptoms associated with iron deficiency include hair loss, brittle nails, and a weakened immune system. Nevertheless, iron supplementation is not recommended unless a lab test determines that iron deficiency is present.

• *Salicylates and sodium and potassium depletion:* Depletion of sodium and potassium ions can result in muscle weakness, fatigue, dehydration, tetany (muscle spasms), and postural hypotension, which can cause dizziness and fainting spells. Other symptoms associated with potassium depletion include irregular heartbeat, poor reflexes, fatigue, continuous thirst, edema, constipation, mental confusion, and nervous disorders.

• *Salicylates and vitamin B₅ (pantothenic acid) depletion:* Although salicylates have been reported to deplete vitamin B_5, that vitamin is so widely available in foods that deficiency is rare. Experimentally induced deficiencies manifest as problems related to the skin, liver, thymus, and nerves. Fatigue and listlessness also are associated with vitamin B_5 deficiency.

■ SULFASALAZINE

Sulfasalazine has been reported to deplete folic acid.

Folic acid depletion can cause a wide range of health problems including anemia, depression, and elevated homocysteine, which is a risk factor for cardiovascular disease. Folic acid deficiency also increases the risk for breast and colorectal cancers. Women who become deficient in folic acid are at greater risk for producing children with birth defects and of developing cervical dysplasia. (For a detailed discussion of folic acid deficiency problems (see pages 50–51.)

■ INDOMETHACIN

Indomethacin has been reported to cause a depletion of folic acid and iron.

• *Indomethacin and folic acid depletion:* Folic acid depletion can cause a wide range of health problems including anemia, depression, and elevated homocysteine, which is a serious risk factor for cardiovascular disease. Folic acid deficiency also increases the risk for developing breast and colorectal cancers. Women who become deficient in folic acid put the fetus at greater risk for birth defects, and the pregnant woman for developing cervical dysplasia. (For a detailed discussion of folic acid deficiency problems, see pages 50–51.

• *Indomethacin and iron depletion:* Iron depletion can cause anemia, which produces weakness and fatigue. Other symptoms associated with iron deficiency include hair loss, brittle nails, and a weakened immune system. Nevertheless, iron supplementation is not recommended unless a lab test determines the presence of iron deficiency.

■ OTHER NON-STEROIDAL ANTI-INFLAMMATORY DRUGS (NSAIDS)

NSAIDs deplete folic acid.

The NSAID classification was extremely successful when these drugs were sold as prescription drugs. Now that NSAIDs are available without a prescription, the concern is greater because people can use the drugs without monitoring by physicians or pharmacists.

Non-steroidal anti-inflammatory drugs showed remarkable sales growth in 2000, totaling $9.5 billion, or 3% of all global pharmaceutical sales.[7] Pharmacia's Celebrex® and Merck's Vioxx®, the two leading COX-2 inhibitors, have had exceptional sales success. Celebrex secured the lead product position after just 11 months on the market. By the end of 2000, it had captured 25% of the world market, with sales growth of 65%. Vioxx was the second best-selling antirheumatic non-steroidal product in 2000, comprising 19.1% of the worldwide market with sales growth of 363%. The leading older NSAIDs all have experienced declining sales in 2000 as a result of the launch of the COX-2 inhibitors, a new class of NSAIDs.

Folic acid deficiency poses greater risks for women than men because of the link to cervical dysplasia, as well as birth defects in their children. Other problems associated with folic acid depletion include anemia, depression, elevated homocysteine (a risk factor for cardiovascular disease) and increased risks for developing breast and colorectal cancers. (For a more detailed description of folic acid deficiency problems, see pages 50–51.

ANTI-PARKINSON'S DISEASE DRUG: LEVODOPA

Parkinson's disease is an inflammatory disease that affects dopamine receptor activity, leading to a variety of symptoms including loss of voluntary muscle control, fatigue, and immune system alterations.

Levodopa depletes potassium, SAMe, and vitamin B_6.

* *Levodopa depletes potassium:* Potassium depletion can produce symptoms of muscular weakness, tetany (muscle spasms), and postural hypotension (low blood pressure when changing from a lying or sitting position to a standing position), which can result in dizziness and fainting spells. Other symptoms associated with potassium depletion include irregular heartbeat, poor reflexes, fatigue, continuous thirst, edema, constipation, mental confusion, and nervous disorders.

* *Levodopa depletes SAMe:* SAMe plays a key role in several important biochemical pathways involving the synthesis of DNA and RNA, phospholipids, proteins, and various neurotransmitters. SAMe deficiency increases the risk for cardiovascular disease, liver disease, depression, insomnia, and estrogen metabolism alterations.

* *Levodopa depletes vitamin B_6:* Depletion of vitamin B_6 can result in depression and insomnia, as well as pose an increased risk for cardiovascular disease. For a detailed discussion of vitamin B_6 depletion problems, see pages 56–57.

ANTIPROTOZOALS: PENTAMIDINE

The prevalence of protazoal infections is becoming more and more recognized. As more physicians investigate these type of infections in their patients, the use of the use of these drugs will increase.

Pentamidine depletes magnesium.

Pentamidine, which usually is used with HIV and AIDS patients to help prevent opportunistic infections, can cause a severe loss of magnesium. In turn, magnesium depletion can produce cardiac arrhythmias and palpitation, hypertension (high blood pressure), and various other cardiovascular-related problems. Additional conditions associated with low magnesium levels include osteoporosis, muscle cramps and muscular weakness, PMS, anxiety, nervousness, insomnia, and increased frequency and severity of asthma attacks.

ANTIVIRAL DRUGS

The antiviral drugs discussed here are the reverse transcriptase inhibitors and a single drug named foscarnet. Most of the research with reverse transcriptase inhibitors regarding nutrient depletions has been done with zidovudine (AZT). Other related drugs that may cause similar nutrient depletions include didanosine, lamivudine, stavudine, zalcitabine, delavirdine, and nevirapine.

■ REVERSE TRANSCRIPTASE INHIBITORS: ZIDOVUDINE (AZT)
AND RELATED DRUGS

Zidovudine (AZT) depletes vitamin B_{12}, copper, zinc, and L-carnitine.

• *Zidovudine and vitamin B_{12} depletion:* A deficiency of vitamin B_{12} can cause anemia, accompanied by tiredness, weakness, and fatigue. Inadequate vitamin B_{12} also can produce elevated levels of homocysteine, which is a risk factor for cardiovascular disease. Long-term B_{12} deficiency can result in permanent nerve damage. Another common manifestation of vitamin B_{12} deficiency is depression, especially in elderly people.

• *Zidovudine and copper depletion:* Copper depletion can cause anemia and fatigue, problems with maintenance and repair of connective tissues, and elevated levels of serum cholesterol.

• *Zidovudine and zinc depletion:* Zinc is an important mineral for a healthy immune system and is needed for the maturation of T killer cells. Zinc deficiency can cause slow-healing of wounds and a weakened immune system, as well as a loss of the senses of taste and smell. Zinc deficiency also can cause infertility and sexual dysfunction in men and women. It is somewhat of a paradox that a drug like this is given to AIDS patients, who have weakened immunity and require immune support, yet zidovudine depletes zinc, which weakens the immune system.

• **Zidovudine and carnitine depletion:** Carnitine is an amino acid that facilitates the transport of fats across cellular membranes for metabolism and the production of energy. Although the body normally produces adequate levels of carnitine, the administration of zidovudine can create a carnitine deficiency, which can result in fatigue, muscle weakness, and cramps.

■ FOSCARNET

Foscarnet is used primarily to prevent opportunistic infections in individuals with HIV.

Foscarnet depletes calcium, magnesium, and potassium.

• **Foscarnet and calcium depletion:** A low level of calcium is one of the primary side effects of taking foscarnet. Calcium depletion can result in skeletal problems such as osteoporosis and osteomalacia. Calcium deficiency also can also cause high blood pressure, muscle cramps, heart palpitation, tooth decay, back and leg pains, insomnia, and nervous disorders.

• **Foscarnet and magnesium depletion:** Magnesium depletion can produce cardiac arrhythmias, high blood pressure, and various other cardiovascular-related problems. Additional conditions associated with low magnesium levels include osteoporosis, muscle cramps, PMS, and an increase in the frequency and severity of asthma attacks.

• **Foscarnet and potassium depletion:** Potassium depletion can cause symptoms of muscular weakness, tetany (muscle spasms), and postural hypotension (low blood pressure when changing from a lying or sitting position to a standing position), which can produce dizziness and fainting spells. Other symptoms associated with potassium depletion include irregular heartbeat, poor reflexes, fatigue, continuous thirst, edema, constipation, mental confusion, and nervous disorders.

BRONCHODILATORS

Bronchodialators help the bronchioles of the lungs to expand and take in more oxygen. These drugs are commonly used in treating asthma. The bronchodilators include theophylline-containing drugs and the beta$_2$ adrenergic agonists (Albuterol®, Terbutaline®).

■ THEOPHYLLINE

Theophylline depletes vitamin B$_6$ (pyridoxine).

- *Theophylline and vitamin B_6 (pyridoxine) depletion:* Depletion of vitamin B_6 can bring about depression and insomnia, and it poses an increased risk for cardiovascular disease.

  - *Depression:* Pyridoxine is necessary for conversion of the amino acid tryptophan into the neurotransmitter serotonin. A deficiency of serotonin in the brain is strongly associated with depression. Therefore, people taking drugs that deplete vitamin B_6 are at greater risk for depression.

  - *Insomnia:* In the brain, serotonin is converted into melatonin, a hormone that controls sleep. Because a vitamin B_6 deficiency inhibits the synthesis of serotonin, it also decreases the amount of melatonin that can be produced in the brain. People who become deficient in melatonin have insomnia and related sleep problems.

  - *Cardiovascular disease:* Vitamin B_6 is one of the B vitamins necessary to metabolize homocysteine, an amino acid produced from metabolism of the essential amino acid methionine. Homocysteine is a toxic substance capable of directly injuring the lining of the arteries, leading to atherosclerosis. Under normal conditions, homocysteine exists only a short time, but a lack of vitamin B_6 results in elevated levels of homocysteine in the blood. Even slight elevations of homocysteine represent a seriously increased risk for developing atherosclerosis, which is the leading cause of heart disease.

■ BETA$_2$ ADRENERGIC AGONISTS

Beta$_2$ adrenergic agonists, which include Albuterol® and Terbutaline®, deplete potassium.

- Potassium depletion can produce muscular weakness, tetany (muscle spasms), and postural hypotension (low blood pressure when changing from a lying or sitting position to a standing position), which can cause dizziness and fainting spells. Other symptoms associated with potassium depletion are irregular heartbeat, poor reflexes, fatigue, continuous thirst, edema, constipation, mental confusion, and nervous disorders. In a hospital setting, symptoms usually are treated and managed by giving intravenous potassium chloride.

CARDIOVASCULAR DRUGS

The classes of cardiovascular drugs are ACE inhibitors, beta-blockers, calcium channel blockers, cardiac glycosides, clonidine and methyldopa, hydralazine-containing vasodilators, loop diuretics, potassium-sparing diuretics, and thiazide diuretics. Each of these will be discussed along with their nutrient depletions.

■ ACE INHIBITORS

In 2001, ACE inhibitors comprised the fourth largest dollar-volume category of prescription drugs in the United States, accounting for more than 101 million prescriptions written for these agents. This represents 3.2% of the total market of prescription drugs.[7]

ACE Inhibitors deplete zinc.

• **ACE inhibitors and zinc depletion:** The mineral zinc is important to the immune system. A zinc deficiency can cause slow healing of wounds and a weakened immune system. A zinc deficiency also can produce insulin resistance, a loss of the senses of taste and smell, and infertility and sexual dysfunction in men and women alike.

■ BETA-BLOCKERS

In 2001, beta-blockers represented the fifth largest category of prescription drugs in the United States, with more than 97 million prescriptions written. This represents 3% of the total prescription drug market.[8]

Beta-blockers deplete coenzyme Q_{10} and melatonin.

• **Beta-blockers and coenzyme Q_{10} depletion:** Beta-blockers comprise just one of numerous classes of drugs that deplete coenzyme Q_{10}, a nutrient that is an extremely important antioxidant and also performs a vital role in generating energy in the mitochondria of all cells. Because the heart is the most active muscle in the human body, a decline in energy resulting from a deficiency of CoQ_{10} first affects the heart, and now it is thought that a CoQ_{10} deficiency may be one of the primary causes of congestive heart failure. In addition to providing antioxidant protection within the mitochondria, CoQ_{10} protects LDL-cholesterol from free radical oxidation. Individuals who are deficient in CoQ_{10} are at increased risk for cardiovascular disease and also have more free radical damage, which accelerates the aging process. CoQ_{10} depletion also causes muscular weakness and may effect blood sugar regulation.

• **Beta-blockers and melatonin depletion:** The beta-blockers propranolol, atenolol, and metaprolol have been found to inhibit the synthesis and release of melatonin, the brain hormone that triggers or induces sleep. A deficiency of melatonin results in insomnia and related sleep problems. Insomnia can lead to many other problems such as depression, poor performance at work, and an increase in accidents. Melatonin also is an important antioxidant, so a depletion of melatonin could result in more free radical damage and an acceleration of the aging process. Finally, many studies have associated low levels of melatonin with an increased incidence of breast cancer.

■ CALCIUM CHANNEL BLOCKERS: NIFEDIPINE AND VERAPAMIL

In 2001, calcium channel blockers comprised the sixth largest category in terms of number of prescriptions written, 94 million. This represented 2.9% of the prescription drug market. Sales of *calcium antagonists, plain,* the fourth-largest therapy class in the world market, grew 2%, to $9.8 billion, or 3.1% of all global pharmaceutical sales in 2000. Pfizer's Norvasc was the leading product in this class worldwide, increasing its market share to 34% in 2000 from 30.2% in 1999.[9]

Nifedipine and verapamil cause potassium depletion (hypokalemia).

• **Nifedipine and verapamil and potassium depletion:** Some of the cardiovascular side effects associated with nifedipine and verapamil stem from potassium depletion. The insufficiency of this mineral can cause symptoms of muscular weakness, tetany (muscle spasms), and postural hypotension (low blood pressure when changing from a lying or sitting position to a standing position), which can cause dizziness and fainting spells. Other symptoms associated with potassium deficiency are irregular heartbeat, poor reflexes, fatigue, continuous thirst, edema, constipation, mental confusion, and nervous disorders.

■ CARDIAC GLYCOSIDES: DIGOXIN

Digoxin causes the depletion of calcium, magnesium, phosphorus, and vitamin B_1.

• **Cardiac glycosides and calcium depletion:** Digoxin increases urinary calcium excretion. To maintain adequate calcium in the blood, the body begins leaching calcium out of the bones, which can result in skeletal problems such as osteoporosis and osteomalacia. Calcium deficiency also can cause high blood pressure, muscle cramps, heart palpitation, tooth decay, back and leg pains, insomnia, and nervous disorders.

• **Cardiac glycosides and magnesium depletion:** Digoxin reduces the reabsorption of magnesium in the kidneys, which increases the urinary excretion of magnesium. Low magnesium levels produce a wide variety of clinical symptoms, including irregular heartbeat and, palpitation high blood pressure, and various other cardiovascular-related problems. Additional conditions associated with low magnesium levels include osteoporosis, muscle cramps and muscular weakness, PMS, anxiety, nervousness, insomnia, fatigue, and an increase in the frequency and severity of asthma attacks.

• **Cardiac glycosides and phosphorus depletion:** Digoxin causes increased urinary excretion of phosphorus. A phosphorus deficiency can cause symptoms such as anxiety and nervousness, as well as skeletal problems.

- **Cardiac glycosides and vitamin B₁ depletion:** Digoxin depletes cellular thiamin and also hinders the cells' ability to incorporate thiamin. This vitamin B₁ deficiency can cause depression, irritability, memory loss, muscle weakness, and edema.

■ CENTRALLY ACTING ANTIHYPERTENSIVE AGENTS: CLONIDINE AND METHYLDOPA

Centrally acting antihypertensive agents exert their effects by acting on centers within the brain that regulate blood pressure.

Clonidine and methyldopa deplete coenzyme Q_{10}.

- **Clonidine and methyldopa deplete coenzyme Q_{10}:** Coenzyme Q_{10} is an extremely important antioxidant and also performs vital roles in generating energy in the mitochondria of all cells. Because the heart is the most active muscle in the human body, a decline in energy resulting from a deficiency of CoQ_{10} first affects the heart, and now it is thought that a CoQ_{10} deficiency may be one of the primary causes of congestive heart failure. In addition to providing antioxidant protection within the mitochondria, CoQ_{10} protects LDL-cholesterol from free radical oxidation. Individuals who are deficient in CoQ_{10} are at increased risk for cardiovascular disease and also have more free radical damage, which accelerates the aging process. Additional effects are muscle weakness and problems with blood sugar regulation.

■ HYDRALAZINE-CONTAINING VASODILATORS

Hydralazine-containing vasodilators deplete vitamin B_6 and coenzyme Q_{10}.

- **Hydralazine-containing vasodilators and vitamin B_6 depletion:** Depletion of vitamin B_6 (pyridoxine) can cause depression and insomnia and puts the person at increased risk for cardiovascular disease.

  - *Depression:* Vitamin B_6 is necessary for converting the amino acid tryptophan into the neurotransmitter serotonin. A deficiency of serotonin in the brain is strongly associated with depression. Therefore, people taking drugs that deplete vitamin B_6 are at greater risk for developing depression.

  - *Insomnia:* In the brain, serotonin is converted into melatonin, a hormone that controls sleep. Because a vitamin B_6 deficiency inhibits the synthesis of serotonin, it also decreases the amount of melatonin that can be produced in the brain. People who become deficient in melatonin will have insomnia and related sleep problems.

  - *Cardiovascular disease:* Vitamin B_6 is one of the B vitamins necessary to metabolize homocysteine, an amino acid produced from the metabolism of the essential amino acid methionine. Homocysteine is a toxic substance capable of directly injuring the lining of the arteries, which is the type of damage that causes atherosclerosis. Under normal conditions homocysteine exists only briefly. A lack of vitamin B_6, however, results only elevated levels of homocysteine in the blood. Even slight elevations of homocysteine represent a seriously increased risk for developing atherosclerosis, the leading cause of heart disease.

• *Hydralazine and coenzyme Q_{10} depletion:* Coenzyme Q_{10} is an extremely important antioxidant and also performs a vital role in generating energy in the mitochondria of all cells. Because the heart is the most active muscle in the human body, a decline in energy resulting from a deficiency of Q_{10} first affects the heart, and it is now thought that a Q_{10} deficiency may be one of the primary causes of congestive heart failure. In addition to providing antioxidant protection within the mitochondria, coenzyme Q_{10} protects LDL-cholesterol from free radical oxidation. Individuals who are deficient in coenzyme Q_{10} are at increased risk for cardiovascular disease and also have more free radical damage, which accelerates the aging process. Additional effects are muscular weakness and problems with blood sugar regulation.

■ LOOP DIURETICS

Loop diuretics cause a depletion of calcium, magnesium, potassium, vitamin B_1, vitamin B_6, vitamin C, sodium, and zinc.

• *Loop diuretics and calcium depletion:* Loop diuretics cause excessive urinary excretion of calcium. To maintain adequate calcium in the blood, the body begins to leach calcium out of the bones, which can result in skeletal problems such as osteoporosis and osteomalacia. Calcium deficiency also can also cause high blood pressure, muscle cramps, heart palpitation, tooth decay, back and leg pains, insomnia, and nervous disorders.

• *Loop diuretics and magnesium depletion:* Loop diuretics cause excessive excretion of magnesium in the urine. Magnesium depletion can produce cardiac arrhythmias and palpitation, high blood pressure, and various other cardiovascular-related problems. Additional conditions associated with low magnesium levels include osteoporosis, muscle cramps and muscular weakness, PMS, insomnia, anxiety, nervousness, and increased frequency and severity of asthma attacks.

• *Loop diuretics and potassium depletion:* Loop diuretics increase the urinary excretion of potassium, which may lead to hypokalemia (potassium depletion). Symptoms are muscular weakness, tetany (muscle spasms), and postural hypotension (low blood pressure when changing from a lying or sitting position to a standing position), which can precipitate dizziness and fainting spells. Other symptoms associated with potassium depletion are irregular heartbeat, poor reflexes, fatigue, continuous thirst, edema, constipation, mental confusion, and nervous disorders.

• *Loop diuretics and vitamin B₁ (thiamin) depletion:* Vitamin B_1 deficiency is a relatively common consequence of taking loop diuretics. Vitamin B_1 deficiency can cause depression, irritability, memory loss, muscle weakness, and edema. In one study, the authors noted that administration of vitamin B_1 resulted in improvement in both verbal and nonverbal IQ scores.

• *Loop diuretics and vitamin B₆ (pyridoxine) depletion:* Loop diuretics can cause substantial urinary loss of pyridoxine. A deficiency of pyridoxine (vitamin B_6) is associated with depression, insomnia, and increased risk for cardiovascular disease.

– *Depression,* Vitamin B_6 is necessary for conversion of the amino acid tryptophan into the neurotransmitter serotonin. A deficiency of serotonin in the brain is strongly associated with depression. Therefore, people taking drugs that deplete vitamin B_6 are at greater risk for depression.

– *Insomnia:* In the brain, serotonin is converted into melatonin, a hormone that controls sleep. Because a vitamin B_6 deficiency inhibits the synthesis of serotonin, it also will decrease the amount of melatonin that can be produced in the brain. People who are deficient in melatonin have insomnia and related sleep problems.

– *Cardiovascular disease:* Vitamin B_6 is one of the B vitamins necessary to metabolize homocysteine, an amino acid produced from metabolism of the essential amino acid methionine. Homocysteine is a toxic substance capable of directly injuring the lining of the arteries, which leads to atherosclerosis. Under normal conditions, homocysteine exists only briefly. A lack of vitamin B_6, results in an elevated level of homocysteine in the blood. Even a slight elevation of homocysteine poses a serious risk factor for developing atherosclerosis, the leading cause of heart disease.

• *Loop diuretics and vitamin C depletion:* Increased urinary excretion of vitamin C begins within 3 hours after taking a dose of a loop diuretic. Vitamin C deficiency can result in a substantially weakened immune system and more free radical damage, which accelerates the aging process.

• *Loop diuretics and sodium depletion:* Sodium depletion is the mechanism of action of loop diuretics, therefore, sodium replacement is *not* appropriate. Nevertheless, too high a dose could cause excessive sodium depletion, which could produce symptoms including muscle weakness, dehydration, loss of appetite, and poor concentration.

• *Loop diuretics and zinc depletion:* Zinc is important to a healthy immune system. Zinc deficiency can cause slow healing of wounds, a weakened immune system, decreased sperm motility, and infertility and sexual dysfunction in men and women alike. Zinc deficiency also can result in a loss of the senses of taste and smell.

■ POTASSIUM-SPARING DIURETICS

Potassium-sparing diuretics deplete calcium, folic acid, and zinc.

• *Potassium-sparing diuretics and calcium depletion:* Potassium-sparing diuretics cause a significant increase in urinary calcium excretion. To maintain adequate calcium in the blood, the body begins leaching calcium out of the bones, which can result in the skeletal problems such as osteoporosis and osteomalacia. Calcium deficiency also can cause high blood pressure, muscle cramps, heart palpitation, tooth decay, back and leg pains, insomnia, and nervous disorders.

• *Potassium-sparing diuretics and folic acid depletion:* The active ingredient in potassium-sparing diuretics is triamterene. Triamterene is classified as a folic acid antagonist, which means that it inhibits the conversion of folic acid to its active form in the body. A folic acid deficiency can result in numerous health problems, especially in women, and folic acid needs are greater during pregnancy. Folic acid insufficiency disrupts DNA metabolism, which causes the production of abnormal cells. This problem is especially acute in cells with the most rapid rates of turnover — red blood cells, white blood cells, and epithelial cells of the stomach, intestine, vagina, and uterine cervix.

Insufficient folic acid also is one of the most common vitamin deficiencies. In addition to people not eating enough green leafy vegetables, folic acid is easily destroyed by heat, light, and oxygen, and substantial losses occur during food processing, cooking, and storage.

Folic acid deficiency can cause anemia, birth defects, cervical dysplasia, elevated homocysteine, headache, fatigue, depression, hair loss, anorexia, insomnia, diarrhea, nausea, and increased infections. Folic acid deficiency also is associated with increased risk for breast cancer and colorectal cancer. The major folic acid deficiency-related health problems are described briefly below.

– *Anemia:* Folic acid is required for the production of erythrocytes (red blood cells), which carry oxygen from the lungs to the tissues and carbon dioxide from the tissues to the lungs. Folic acid deficiency causes anemia and reduced tissue oxygenation. This results in a condition known as megaloblastic anemia, with symptoms of tiredness, weakness, diarrhea, and weight loss.

- *Birth defects:* Folic acid helps regulate neural development and the transfer of genetic material to new cells in the fetus. During pregnancy, the rapidly growing fetus substantially increases the woman's need for folic acid, and folic acid deficiency during pregnancy dramatically increases the risk of birth defects such as spina bifida and cleft palate. The link between folic acid deficiency and birth defects is so strong that all women of childbearing age are advised to have their folic acid status checked before trying to become pregnant. If this practice were followed, thousands of birth defects probably would be prevented each year. A laboratory test, the Neutrophilic Hypersegmentation Index (NHI), easily identifies folic acid insufficiency.

- *Cervical dysplasia:* The development of abnormal cells in the uterus, cervical dysplasia, is regarded as a precancerous condition that usually is discovered when a woman has a Pap exam. This condition may contribute to an increased number of hysterectomies. Approximately 800,000 women have hysterectomies every year in the United States. Some health-care professionals believe that the folic acid depletion caused by oral contraceptives and other medications is linked to this high incidence of cervical dysplasia and hysterectomies.

- *Elevated homocysteine,* also known as hyperhomocysteinemia, is recognized as a serious independent risk factor for cardiovascular disease. Excess homocysteine is can cause direct damage to vascular endothelial cells, the type of damage that initiates plaque build-up in the arteries. Even moderate elevations of homocysteine represent substantially increased risk for the development of plaque build-up and blood clots.

• *Potassium-sparing diuretics and zinc depletion:* Triamterene, the primary ingredient in potassium-sparing diuretics, causes increased urinary excretion of zinc. Zinc is extremely important to the immune system. Thus, zinc deficiency can cause slow wound-healing and a weakened immune system. Other zinc deficiency problems include loss of the senses of taste and smell, decreased sperm motility, and infertility and sexual dysfunction in men and women alike.

■ THIAZIDE DIURETICS

Thiazide diuretics deplete coenzyme Q_{10}, magnesium, potassium, sodium, and zinc.

• *Thiazide diuretics and coenzyme Q_{10} depletion:* Coenzyme Q_{10} is an extremely important antioxidant and also performs vital roles in generating energy in the mitochondria of all cells. Because the heart is the most active muscle in the human body, a decline in energy arising from a deficiency of CoQ_{10} first affects the heart, and now it is thought that a CoQ_{10} deficiency might be one of the primary causes of congestive heart failure. In addition to providing antioxidant protection within the mitochondria, CoQ_{10} protects LDL-cholesterol from free radical oxidation. It also plays a role in blood sugar regulation. Individuals who are deficient in CoQ_{10} are at increased risk for cardiovascular disease and also will incur more free radical damage, which accelerates the aging process. An additional symptom of CoQ_{10} depletion is muscle weakness.

• *Thiazide diuretics and magnesium depletion:* Thiazide diuretics cause excess magnesium to be lost in the urine. Low magnesium levels are known to produce a wide variety of clinical symptoms, including irregular heartbeat, high blood pressure, and various other cardiovascular-related problems. Additional conditions associated with low magnesium levels include osteoporosis, muscle cramps, PMS, and an increase in the frequency and severity of asthma attacks.

• *Thiazide diuretics and potassium depletion:* Thiazide diuretics cause increased urinary excretion of potassium, which may lead to hypokalemia (potassium depletion). This can produce symptoms of muscular weakness, tetany (muscle spasms), and postural hypotension (low blood pressure when changing from a lying or sitting position to a standing position), which can cause fainting spells. Other symptoms associated with potassium depletion are irregular heartbeat, poor reflexes, fatigue, continuous thirst, edema, constipation, mental confusion, and nervous disorders.

• *Thiazide diuretics and sodium depletion:* Sodium depletion is the mechanism of action of thiazide diuretics, therefore, sodium replacement is *not* appropriate. Too high a dose, however, could cause excessive sodium depletion. Symptoms associated with sodium insufficiency include muscle weakness, dehydration, loss of appetite, and poor concentration.

• *Thiazide diuretics and zinc depletion:* Thiazide diuretics cause a substantial increase in urinary output of zinc. Zinc is extremely important to the immune system, and a zinc deficiency can cause a weakened immune system as well as slow healing of wounds. Zinc deficiency also can result in a loss of the senses of taste and smell, decreased sperm motility and infertility and sexual dysfunction in men and women alike.

CHEMOTHERAPY DRUGS

Many of the drugs used to treat cancer can cause multiple nutrient depletions through several different mechanisms. Some of these drugs damage the cells lining the intestinal tract, which inhibits the absorption of nutrients. Damage to these cells also creates inflammation and pain, which becomes more intense when food and digestives juices come into contact with the damaged cells. Ulceration in the mouth and throat also may develop.

Frequently, cancer patients lose their appetite because eating is too painful, and this contributes to nutrient depletions. Many chemotherapy medications also incite nausea, diarrhea, and vomiting, which can exacerbate nutrient depletions. Administration of intravenous vitamins and minerals can be helpful to cancer patients who are too sick to eat properly and absorb nutrients.

CHOLESTEROL-LOWERING DRUGS

The four classes of cholesterol-lowering drugs are: (1) the HMG-CoA reductase inhibitors (the statins), (2) the bile acid sequesterants, (3) the "fibrates," which include clofibrate and fenofibrate, and (4) gemfibrozil, an individual cholesterol-lowering drug that does not fit into either of the other categories.

■ HMG-COA REDUCTASE INHIBITORS (THE STATINS)

Sales of cholesterol and triglyceride reducers — drugs used to reduce cholesterol in the bloodstream — grew 21% in 2000, placing this class second in total world sales. The statin drugs (atorvastatin, simvastatin, lovastatin, and others) dominated this class in 2000. Pfizer's Lipitor assumed the lead position, generating 40% growth and 33.8% market share.[10]

Statin drugs deplete coenzyme Q_{10}.

The "statin" drugs, also known as HMG-CoA reductase inhibitors, represent one of numerous classes of drugs that deplete coenzyme Q_{10}, an extremely important antioxidant that also performs vital roles in generating energy in the mitochondria of all cells. Because the heart is the most active muscle in the human body, a decline in energy resulting from a deficiency of CoQ_{10} first affects the heart, and now it is thought that a CoQ_{10} deficiency might be one of the main causes of congestive heart failure.

In addition to providing antioxidant protection within the mitochondria, CoQ_{10} protects LDL-cholesterol from free radical oxidation. Individuals who are deficient in coenzyme CoQ_{10} are at increased risk for cardiovascular disease, muscular weakness, and alterations in blood sugar regulation, and the deficiency also produces more free radical damage, which accelerates the aging process.

■ BILE ACID SEQUESTRANTS

The two drugs in this class of cholesterol-lowering medication are cholestyramine and colestipol. Because these drugs are seldom used these days, the nutrient depletions associated with them are summarized instead of discussing each nutrient depletion separately. These drugs function by inhibiting the absorption of cholesterol in the intestines. In doing so, however, they inhibit the absorption of many other nutrients. Individuals who are taking one of these drugs are urged to take nutritional supplements several hours before taking a dose of the medication, which will give the nutrients a better chance of being absorbed before the medication arrives in the intestines.

The bile acid sequestrants deplete fat-soluble vitamins and other vitamins.

• Cholestyramine depletes all of the fat-soluble vitamins, which include vitamins A, D, E, and K. Other nutrients that are depleted are vitamin B_{12}, folic acid, beta-carotene, and the minerals calcium, iron, magnesium, phosphorus, and zinc.

• Colestipol depletes the fat-soluble vitamins, including vitamins A, D, E, and K. Other nutrients that are depleted include beta-carotene, folic acid, vitamin B_{12}, and iron.

■ THE FIBRATES

The "fibrates," which include clofibrate and fenofibrate, deplete vitamin E, vitamin B_{12}, copper, and zinc.

• *Clofibrate and fenofibrate deplete vitamin E:* Vitamin E is one of the body's most important antioxidant nutrients. A deficiency of vitamin E results in more free radical damage, which accelerates the aging process. One of the most immediate consequences of vitamin E depletion is increased oxidation of LDL-cholesterol, which speeds up the process of atherosclerosis.

• *Clofibrate and fenofibrate deplete vitamin B_{12}:* Vitamin B_{12} deficiency can cause anemia, which results in fatigue, tiredness, and weakness, and B_{12} deficiency is a common cause of depression, especially in elderly people. Inadequate B_{12} also causes elevated homocysteine, which poses a seriously increased risk for cardiovascular disease. If serious B_{12} deficiencies are not corrected, long-term irreversible neurological damage can occur.

• *Clofibrate and fenofibrate deplete copper:* Copper depletion can result in anemia and fatigue, problems with the maintenance and repair of connective tissues, and elevated levels of serum cholesterol.

• *Clofibrate and fenofibrate deplete zinc:* Zinc is important to a healthy immune system. Indications of a zinc deficiency are slow healing of wounds and a weakened immune system. Other zinc deficiency problems include insulin resistance, a loss of the senses of taste and smell, and infertility and sexual dysfunction in both men and women.

■ GEMFIBROZIL

Gemfibrozil depletes coenzyme Q_{10}, vitamin E, and gamma tocopherol.

Although it effectively improves blood cholesterol, gemfibrozil reportedly causes a 41.5% decline in coenzyme Q_{10}, a 39.7% decline in vitamin E (alpha tocopherol), and a 50% decline in gamma tocopherol (another form of vitamin E, with anti-cancer properties).[11]

• *Gemfibrozil and coenzyme Q_{10} depletion:* Coenzyme Q_{10} is an extremely important antioxidant and also performs vital roles in generating energy in the mitochondria of all cells. Because the heart is the most active muscle in the human body, a decline in energy resulting from a deficiency of CoQ_{10} first affects the heart, and now it is thought that a CoQ_{10} deficiency may be one of the primary causes of congestive heart failure. In addition to providing antioxidant protection within the mitochondria, CoQ_{10} protects LDL-cholesterol from free radical oxidation. Individuals who are deficient in CoQ_{10} are at increased risk for cardiovascular disease and also have more free radical damage, which accelerates the aging process. Additional effects are muscular weakness and problems with blood sugar regulation.

• *Gemfibrozil and vitamin E depletion:* Vitamin E is one of the body's most important antioxidant nutrients. A deficiency of vitamin E results in free radical damage, which accelerates the aging process. One of the most immediate consequences of vitamin E depletion is increased oxidation of LDL-cholesterol, which speeds up the process of atherosclerosis.

• *Gemfibrozil and gamma tocopherol depletion:* Gamma tocopherol is a form of vitamin E that also has fat-soluble antioxidant properties. Gamma tocopherol actually may provide stronger anticancer activity than the alpha tocopherol form of vitamin E. Thus, the depletion of gamma tocopherol might weaken the portion of an individual's immune system that protects against cancer.

ELECTROLYTE REPLACEMENT: TIMED-RELEASE POTASSIUM CHLORIDE

Several categories of drugs deplete potassium. Potassium chloride is prescribed for restoring potassium levels.

Timed-release potassium chloride medications cause a depletion of Vitamin B_{12}.

Timed release potassium chloride medications make the ileal section of the intestinal tract more acidic, which inhibits the absorption of vitamin B_{12}. Vitamin B_{12} deficiency can cause anemia, accompanied by fatigue, tiredness, and weakness, and B_{12} deficiency is a common cause of depression, especially in elderly people. Inadequate B_{12} also results in elevated homocysteine, which poses a seriously increased risk for cardiovascular disease. If serious B_{12} deficiencies are not corrected, long-term irreversible neurological damage can occur.

FEMALE HORMONES

The two main categories of female hormones are oral contraceptives, which are used for birth control, and estrogen replacement therapy (ERT), prescribed for the symptoms of menopause as well as the prevention of osteoporosis and cardiovascular disease. Estrogen replacement therapy is also known as hormone replacement replacement therapy (HRT).

■ ORAL CONTRACEPTIVES

In 2001, oral contraceptives constituted the seventh largest category of prescription drugs in the United States, accounting for more than 82 million prescriptions written, which represented approximately 2.6% of the total prescription drug market.[12]

Oral contraceptives deplete folic acid, vitamin B_6, vitamin B_{12}, vitamin B_1, vitamin B_2, vitamin B_3, vitamin C, vitamin E, and the minerals magnesium, selenium, and zinc.

• *Oral contraceptives and folic acid depletion:* Folic acid depletion can cause some serious health problems, especially in women, and folic acid needs are greater during pregnancy. Folic acid deficiency disrupts DNA metabolism, which disrupts normal cells. This problem is especially acute in cells with the most rapid rates of turnover, including red blood cells, leukocytes, and epithelial cells of the stomach, intestine, vagina, and uterine cervix. Insufficient folic acid also is one of the most common vitamin deficiencies. In addition to people not eating enough green leafy vegetables, folic acid is easily destroyed by heat, light, and oxygen, and substantial losses occur during food processing, cooking, and storage.

Folic acid deficiency can cause anemia, birth defects, cervical dysplasia, elevated homocysteine, headache, fatigue, depression, hair loss, anorexia, insomnia, diarrhea, nausea, and increased infections. Folic acid deficiency also is associated with increased risk for breast cancer and colorectal cancer. The major health problems related to folic acid insufficiency are described briefly below, underlining the importance of people (especially women) taking folic acid supplementation.

– *Anemia:* Folic acid is required for the production of erythrocytes (red blood cells), which carry oxygen from the lungs to the tissues and carbon dioxide from the tissues to the lungs. Folic acid deficiency causes anemia and reduced tissue oxygenation. This results in a condition known as megaloblastic anemia, which produces tiredness, weakness, diarrhea, and weight loss.

- *Birth defects:* Folic acid helps regulate neural development and the transfer of genetic material to new cells in the fetus. During pregnancy, the rapidly growing fetus substantially increases the woman's need for folic acid, and folic acid deficiency during pregnancy dramatically increases the risk of birth defects such as spina bifida and cleft palate. The link between folic acid deficiency and birth defects is so strong, in fact, that all women of childbearing age are advised to have their folic acid status checked before trying to become pregnant. If this practice were followed, thousands of birth defects probably would be prevented each year. A laboratory test, the Neutrophilic Hypersegmentation Index (NHI), easily identifies folic acid insufficiency.

- *Cervical dysplasia:* The development of abnormal cells in the uterus, cervical dysplasia, is a precancerous condition that usually is discovered when a woman has a Pap exam. This condition may contribute to an increased number of hysterectomies. Approximately 800,000 women have hysterectomies every year in the United States. Some health-care professionals believe that the folic acid depletion induced by oral contraceptives and other medications is linked to this high incidence of cervical dysplasia and hysterectomies.

- *Elevated homocysteine:* Also known as hyperhomocysteinemia, elevated homocysteine is recognized as a independent risk factor for cardiovascular disease. Excess homocysteine can cause direct damage to vascular endothelial cells, the type of damage that initiates plaque build-up in the arteries. Even moderate elevations of homocysteine represent substantially increased risks for plaque build-up and blood clots.

• *Oral contraceptives and vitamin B_6 depletion:* Depletion of vitamin B_6 (pyridoxine) can cause depression and insomnia, and it poses an increased risk for cardiovascular disease.

- *Depression:* Vitamin B_6 is necessary to convert the amino acid tryptophan into the neurotransmitter serotonin. A deficiency of serotonin in the brain is strongly associated with depression. Therefore, people taking drugs that deplete vitamin B_6 are at greater risk for depression.

- *Insomnia:* In the brain, serotonin is converted into melatonin, a hormone that controls sleep. Because a vitamin B_6 deficiency inhibits the synthesis of serotonin, it also decreases the amount of melatonin that can be produced in the brain. People who become deficient in melatonin will incur insomnia and related sleep problems.

– *Cardiovascular disease:* Vitamin B_6 is one of the B vitamins that are necessary to metabolize homocysteine, an amino acid produced from the metabolism of the essential amino acid methionine. Homocysteine is a toxic substance capable of directly injuring the lining of the arteries, the type of damage that causes atherosclerosis. Under normal conditions, it exists only briefly. Insufficiency of vitamin B_6, however, results in elevated homocysteine in the blood. Even slight elevations of homocysteine represent a seriously increased risk for developing atherosclerosis, which is the leading cause of heart disease.

• *Oral contraceptives and vitamin B_{12} depletion:* Vitamin B_{12} deficiency can cause anemia, with accompanying fatigue, tiredness, and weakness, and B_{12} deficiency is a common cause of depression, especially in elderly people. Inadequate B_{12} also causes elevated homocysteine, which poses a seriously increased risk for cardiovascular disease. If serious B_{12} deficiencies are not corrected, long-term irreversible neurological damage can occur.

Note: Oral contraceptives deplete all three of the B-vitamins necessary for metabolism of homocysteine: folic acid, vitamin B_6, and vitamin B_{12}. Deficiency in any one of these vitamins increases homocysteine, which damages the arteries and initiates plaque build-up. The sad part about this scenario is that this is a silent killer. Frequently a person has no symptoms until arteries are more than 90% blocked. This greatly increases the risks for a stroke or a heart attack. Women who are taking oral contraceptives are urged to carefully consider these nutrient depletions and begin taking nutritional supplements now to help prevent serious health problems that could take decades to develop.

• *Oral contraceptives deplete vitamin B_1:* A deficiency of vitamin B_1 can result in depression, irritability, memory loss, muscle weakness, and edema. One study noted that administration of vitamin B_1 to individuals with a B_1 deficiency resulted in improved verbal and nonverbal IQ scores.

• *Oral contraceptives and vitamin B_2 depletion:* Symptoms associated with vitamin B_2 (riboflavin) deficiency include problems with the skin, eyes, mucous membranes, and nerves.

• *Oral contraceptives and vitamin B_3 depletion:* Women have disturbances in the metabolism of tryptophan and outbreaks of pellagra at twice the rate of men. This is presumably because estrogen medications inhibit the conversion of tryptophan to niacin. Niacin deficiency, with pellagra-like symptoms, includes problems with the skin and gastrointestinal and nervous systems.

• *Oral contraceptives and vitamin C depletion:* Vitamin C depletion can result in a weakened immune system. Low levels of vitamin C can accelerate aging damage because of increased free radical damage. In one study, ophthalmologists expressed their concern that vitamin C depletion might increase the risk of developing glaucoma and cataracts.

• *Oral contraceptives and Vitamin E depletion:* Vitamin E is an important fat-soluble antioxidant for the body. Vitamin E reduces the blood "stickiness" that may attend cardiovascular diseases such as atherosclerosis and high cholesterol levels. Vitamin E also helps protect our bodies against cancers and other diseases such as PMS and macular degeneration.

• *Oral contraceptives and tyrosine depletion:* Tyrosine is classified as a nonessential amino acid; however, tyrosine is an essential amino acid because it is part of the structure of almost all proteins in the body. Tyrosine is essential to healthy brain function. It also is a necessary building block in making thyroid hormones, which determine metabolism. Oral contraceptives have been reported to decrease levels of tyrosine in the body.

• *Oral contraceptives and magnesium depletion:* In general, magnesium depletion can cause cardiac arrhythmias, palpitation, high blood pressure and various other cardiovascular-related problems, osteoporosis, anxiety, nervousness, insomnia, muscle weakness, PMS, and an increase in the frequency and severity of asthma attacks.

For women who are taking estrogen-containing medications, the topic of magnesium depletion merits a more detailed explanation. Frequently, the following two factors interact at the same time to increase health problems:

1. Oral contraceptives deplete magnesium.

2. Many women take calcium to prevent osteoporosis.

Taking calcium without extra magnesium magnifies the problems associated with magnesium depletion because calcium and magnesium function as a mineral pair and the relative ratio or balance between these minerals is important. For example, they control the blood-clotting mechanism: Excess calcium increases clotting, and magnesium thins the blood to prevent clotting. They also regulate muscle contraction, in which calcium causes contractions while magnesium works to relax muscles. Thus, the two minerals are counter-regulatory.

Therefore, two factors contribute to, and magnify, the resulting imbalance when women who take oral contraceptives (which deplete magnesium) also take calcium (without magnesium). One of the most frequent side effects associated with oral contraceptives is thrombus (or blood clot) formation.

Now it is clear why this happens: The combination of a depletion of magnesium and an excess of calcium increases the likelihood of clot formation. This also helps to explain why so many women have painful muscle cramps around the time of menstruation every month. Excess calcium increases muscle contraction.

- *Oral contraceptives and selenium depletion:* Selenium is an important antioxidant nutrient. A deficiency of selenium increases the risk for diseases such as cancer and cardiovascular disease. People who are selenium-deficient are subjected to increased free radical damage, which accelerates the aging process.

- *Oral contraceptives and zinc depletion:* Zinc is a mineral that is important to the immune system. A zinc deficiency can cause slow healing of wounds and a weakened immune system. A zinc deficiency also results in insulin resistance, a loss of the senses of taste and smell, and infertility and sexual dysfunction in men and women alike.

■ ESTROGEN REPLACEMENT THERAPY

In 2002, estrogen sales dropped 13% because of the controversy surrounding hormone replacement therapy. Nevertheless, millions of women are still being prescribed and are using estrogen replacement therapy.[13]

A substantial body of research has been published on the nutritional depletions caused by ingesting estrogen in the form of oral contraceptives. Little research has been done, however, on the estrogen-containing medications used for ERT, also referred to as hormone replacement therapy (HRT). To date, studies have reported that orally ingested estrogen medications taken for hormone replacement therapy deplete vitamin B_6 and magnesium. Women should be aware, moreover, that the estrogen-only prescriptions also deplete folic acid, vitamin B_1, vitamin B_2, vitamin B_3, vitamin B_{12}, vitamin C, and zinc.

Hormone replacement therapy deletes vitamin B_6 and magnesium.

- *Estrogen replacement therapy and vitamin B_6 depletion:* Vitamin B_6 (pyridoxine) depletion can lead to depression, insomnia, and an increased risk for cardiovascular disease.

  - *Depression:* Vitamin B_6 is necessary to convert the amino acid tryptophan into the neurotransmitter serotonin. A deficiency of serotonin in the brain is strongly associated with depression. Therefore, people taking drugs that deplete vitamin B_6 are at greater risk for depression.

- *Insomnia:* In the brain, serotonin is converted into melatonin, a hormone that controls sleep. Because a vitamin B_6 deficiency inhibits the synthesis of serotonin, it also decreases the amount of melatonin that can be produced in the brain. People who are deficient in melatonin can have insomnia and related sleep problems.

- *Cardiovascular disease:* Vitamin B_6 is one of the B-vitamins necessary to metabolize homocysteine, an amino acid produced from metabolism of the essential amino acid methionine. Homocysteine is a toxic substance capable of directly injuring the lining of the arteries. This is the type of damage that causes atherosclerosis. Under normal conditions, homocysteine exists only briefly. A lack of vitamin B_6, however, causes elevated homocysteine in the blood, and even slight elevations of homocysteine pose a seriously increased risk for atherosclerosis, the leading cause of heart disease.

• **Estrogen replacement therapy and magnesium depletion:** In general, magnesium depletion can cause cardiac arrhythmias, high blood pressure, heart palpitation and various other cardiovascular-related problems, osteoporosis, muscle cramps, muscle weakness, anxiety, nervousness, insomnia, PMS, and an increase in the frequency and severity of asthma attacks. For women taking estrogen-containing medications, the topic of magnesium depletion deserves a more detailed explanation because frequently two factors happening at the same time interact to increase health problems. First, estrogen replacement therapy medications deplete magnesium. Second, many women take calcium to prevent osteoporosis.

Taking calcium without extra magnesium magnifies the problem of magnesium depletion because calcium and magnesium function as a mineral pair and the relative ratio or balance between these minerals is important. For example, they control the blood-clotting mechanism, and excess calcium increases clotting while magnesium thins the blood to prevent clotting. The two minerals also regulate muscle contraction, in which calcium causes contractions while magnesium works to relax muscles. Thus, they are counter-regulatory.

You can see, then, that two factors contribute to and magnify the imbalance that women who take ERT (which depletes magnesium) who also take calcium (without magnesium) incur. One of the most frequent side effects associated with estrogen-containing medication is thrombus, or blood clot, formation. The depletion of magnesium combined with an excess of calcium increases the likelihood of clot formation. This also helps to explain why so many women have painful muscle cramps around the time of menstruation, because excess calcium increases muscle contraction.

GOUT MEDICATIONS: COLCHICINE

Gout is a condition of inappropriate protein metabolism. Elevations in purine metabolites result in painful inflammation of various joints, particularly in the feet.

Colchicine depletes vitamin B$_{12}$, sodium, potassium, beta-carotene, calcium, and phosphorus.

• *Colchicine and vitamin B$_{12}$ depletion:* A deficiency of vitamin B$_{12}$ can cause anemia, characterized by fatigue, tiredness, and weakness. Insufficient B$_{12}$ also is a common cause of depression, especially in elderly people. Inadequate levels of B$_{12}$ increase homocysteine levels, increasing the risk for cardiovascular disease. If serious B$_{12}$ deficiencies are not corrected, they can lead to long-term irreversible neurological damage.

• *Colchicine and sodium depletion:* Colchicine can cause widespread alteration of intestinal mucus, which hinders intestinal absorption of nutrients and causes increased fecal excretion. Sodium is one of several nutrients reported to be depleted in this manner. Symptoms associated with sodium depletion include muscle weakness, dehydration, loss of appetite, and poor concentration.

• *Colchicine and potassium depletion:* Colchicine can cause widespread alteration of the intestinal mucus, which hinders intestinal absorption of nutrients, causing increased fecal excretion. Potassium is one of several nutrients reported to be depleted in this manner. Loss of potassium can lead to hypokalemia (potassium depletion), accompanied by muscular weakness, tetany (muscle spasms), and postural hypotension (a term that refers to low blood pressure when changing from a lying or sitting position to a standing position), which can induce fainting spells. Other symptoms associated with potassium depletion include irregular heartbeat, poor reflexes, fatigue, continuous thirst, edema, constipation, mental confusion, and nervous disorders.

• *Colchicine and beta-carotene depletion:* Colchicine can cause widespread alteration of the intestinal mucus, which hinders intestinal absorption of nutrients and causes increased fecal excretion. Beta-carotene is one of several nutrients reported to be depleted in this manner.

• *Colchicine and calcium depletion:* Calcium depletion can result in skeletal problems such as osteoporosis and osteomalacia. Calcium deficiency also can cause high blood pressure, muscle cramps, heart palpitation, tooth decay, back and leg pains, insomnia, and nervous disorders.

• *Colchicine and phosphorus depletion:* A phosphorus deficiency can cause symptoms such as anxiety and nervousness, as well as skeletal problems.

LAXATIVES

The three classes of laxatives are those containing mineral oil, bisacodyl, and the phosphate enemas.

■ LAXATIVES CONTAINING MINERAL OIL

Mineral-oil laxatives deplete fat-soluble nutrients, which include vitamins A, D, E, K, and beta-carotene, as well as the minerals calcium and phosphorus.

The following points summarize the various ways in which regular use of mineral oil-containing laxatives can cause the depletion of nutrients.

• Mineral oil is capable of absorbing the fat-soluble vitamins A, D, E, K, and beta-carotene, which prevents them from being absorbed.

• Mineral oil hastens movement of the bowel content, which may prevent complete digestion and absorption of nutrients.

• Mineral oil may interfere with the process of absorption throughout the lower intestines. By partially covering the surface area of the intestines, it establishes a mechanical barrier to absorption and digestion with consequent symptoms of "indigestion."

• Mineral oil interferes with the utilization and retention of calcium and phosphorus. This interference is possibly of a dual nature: (a) Mineral oil interferes with the absorption of these minerals by forming a mechanical barrier along the intestinal tract, and (b) it alters the metabolic processes of calcium and phosphorus by interfering with the absorption of vitamin D.

• Mineral oil mechanically coats food particles and, consequently, prevents their complete absorption through the intestinal walls. This statement is borne out by the fact that the continuous use of mineral oil frequently causes a severe loss in weight.

■ BISACODYL

Bisacodyl causes potassium depletion.

Loss of potassium can lead to hypokalemia (potassium depletion), with symptoms of muscular weakness, tetany (muscle spasms), and postural hypotension (a term that refers to low blood pressure when changing from a lying or sitting position to a standing position), which can cause fainting spells. Other symptoms associated with potassium depletion include irregular heartbeat, poor reflexes, fatigue, continuous thirst, edema, constipation, mental confusion, and nervous disorders.

■ PHOSPHATE ENEMAS

Phosphate enemas deplete calcium and magnesium.

• *Phosphate enemas and calcium depletion:* Calcium depletion can result in skeletal problems such as osteoporosis and osteomalacia. Calcium deficiency also can cause high blood pressure, muscle cramps, heart palpitation, tooth decay, back and leg pains, insomnia, and nervous disorders.

• *Phosphate enemas and magnesium depletion:* Depletion of magnesium can cause cardiac arrhythmias, palpitation, high blood pressure, and various other cardiovascular-related problems. Additional conditions associated with low magnesium levels include osteoporosis, muscle cramps, muscular weakness, PMS, nervousness, insomnia, and an increase in the frequency and severity of asthma attacks.

PSYCHOTHERAPEUTIC DRUGS

The eighth-largest therapy class in 2000 consisted of the antipsychotics, or psychotherapeutic drugs, with worldwide sales of $6 billion. This class represented 1.09% of all global pharmaceutical sales, with a 22% increase in sales over 1999.[14]

The following classes of psychotherapeutic drugs are capable of depleting nutrients in the body: the tricyclic antidepressants, phenothiazines, monoamine oxidase inhibitors (phenelzine and haloperidol), butyrophenones, lithium, and selective serotonin reuptake inhibitors (SSRIs).

■ TRICYCLIC ANTIDEPRESSANTS

Tricyclic antidepressants deplete vitamin B_2 and coenzyme Q_{10}.

• *Tricyclic antidepressants and vitamin B_2 depletion:* Symptoms associated with vitamin B_2 (riboflavin) deficiency include problems with the skin, eyes, mucous membranes, and nerves.

• *Tricyclic antidepressants and coenzyme Q_{10} depletion:* Coenzyme Q_{10} is an extremely important antioxidant and also performs critical roles in the generation of energy in the mitochondria of all cells. CoQ_{10} protects LDL-cholesterol from free radical oxidation. The heart is the most active muscle in the human body, and a decline in energy resulting from a deficiency of CoQ_{10} first affects the heart. Now it is thought that a CoQ_{10} deficiency may be one of the primary causes of congestive heart failure. In short, individuals who are deficient in coenzyme Q_{10} have an increased risk for cardiovascular disease and can have muscle weakness and fatigue, decreased blood sugar regulation, and also have higher levels of free radical damage, which accelerates the aging process.

Some researchers also believe that alterations in CoQ_{10} metabolism can affect the beta cells of the islets of Langerhans in the pancreas. These are the cells that make insulin to control blood sugar. Alterations in blood sugar metabolism can lead to insulin resistance, weight gain, and even diabetes over time.

■ PHENOTHIAZINES

Phenothiazines deplete vitamin B_2, coenzyme Q_{10}, and melatonin.

• *Phenothiazines and vitamin B_2 depletion:* Symptoms associated with vitamin B_2 (riboflavin) deficiency include problems with the skin, eyes, mucous membranes, and nerves.

• *Phenothiazines and coenzyme Q_{10} depletion:* Coenzyme Q_{10} is an extremely important antioxidant and also performs critical roles in the generation of energy in the mitochondria of all cells. Q_{10} protects LDL-cholesterol from free radical oxidation. Because the heart is the most active muscle in the human body, a decline in energy resulting from a deficiency of CoQ_{10} first affects the heart, and now it is thought that a CoQ_{10} deficiency might be one of the main causes of congestive heart failure. Individuals who are deficient in CoQ_{10} are at increased risk for cardiovascular disease, muscular weakness, decreased blood sugar regulation, and accelerated aging as a result of the free radical damage.

• *Phenothiazines and melatonin depletion:* Chlorpromazine depletes melatonin, the brain hormone that triggers or induces sleep. A deficiency of melatonin can result in insomnia and related sleep problems. Insomnia can lead to many other problems such as depression, poor performance at work, increased risk for accidents, decrease in the release of growth hormone, increase in blood sugar dysregulation, and increased inflammatory cytokine activity. Melatonin is also an important antioxidant, so a depletion of melatonin could result in more free radical damage and an acceleration of the aging process. Finally, many studies have associated low levels of melatonin with a higher incidence of breast cancer.

■ MONOAMINE OXIDASE INHIBITORS (MAOIs) (PHENELZINE AND HALOPERIDOL)

Phenelzine depletes vitamin B_6

• *Phenelzine depletes vitamin B_6:* Vitamin B_6 (pyridoxine) depletion can cause depression and insomnia, and it increases the risk for cardiovascular disease. For a more detailed explanation of these vitamin B$_6$-deficiency problems, see pages 56–57.

Haloperidol depletes melatonin and vitamin E.

• *Haloperidol and melatonin depletion:* Melatonin is the brain hormone that triggers or induces sleep. A deficiency results in insomnia and related sleep problems. Insomnia also can lead to depression, poor performance at work, increased risk for accidents, lowered release of growth hormone, increased dysregulation of blood sugar, and increased inflammatory cytokine activity, among other problems. Melatonin is an important antioxidant, so a depletion of melatonin could result in more free radical damage and an acceleration of the aging process. Finally, low levels of melatonin have been associated with an increased incidence of breast cancer.

• *Haloperidol depletes vitamin E:* Vitamin E is one of the body's most important antioxidant nutrients. A deficiency of vitamin E results in more free radical damage, which accelerates the aging process. One of the most immediate consequences of vitamin E depletion is increased oxidation of LDL-cholesterol, which speeds up the process of atherosclerosis.

■ LITHIUM

Lithium depletes inositol.

• *Lithium and inositol depletion:* Lithium reduces brain inositol levels by inhibiting the enzyme inositol monophosphatase. In one study, 80% of patients with bipolar depression who were being treated with lithium were found to have reduced levels of inositol in the brain. Excessive urination and excessive thirst are side effects related to inositol deficiency.

■ SELECTIVE SEROTONIN REUPTAKE INHIBITORS (SSRIs)

To date, no studies support research on drug-induced nutrient depletions for SSRIs.

STEROIDS (ANABOLIC)

Although they are used infrequently in medicine, the principal purpose of steroid use is to stimulate tissue anabolism. Low iron status could retard repair of wounds and reduced oxygenation of tissues.

Stanozolol depletes iron.

• *Stanozolol and iron depletion:* Iron depletion can cause anemia, which produces weakness and fatigue. Other symptoms associated with iron deficiency include hair loss, brittle nails, and a weakened immune system. Nevertheless, iron supplementation is not recommended unless a lab test determines the presence of iron deficiency.

THYROID MEDICATIONS
Levothyroxine depletes iron.

• *Levothyroxine depletes iron:* Iron depletion can cause anemia, which produces weakness and fatigue. Other symptoms associated with iron deficiency include hair loss, brittle nails, and a weakened immune system. However, iron supplementation is not recommended unless a lab test determines that iron deficiency is present.

ULCER MEDICATIONS
In 2000, the anti-ulcer drug class, representing treatments for stomach ulcers, generated $17.4 billion in sales and remains the leading therapeutic class worldwide, as it has for the past 10 years. This class represented 5.5% of all global pharmaceutical sales, with sales rising 13% from 1999. Sales of AstraZeneca's Losec/Prilosec, the world's leading anti-ulcerant product and number-one selling drug across all therapeutic classes, grew 9% year-over-year, to $6.1 billion in 2000.[15]

The two classes of anti-ulcer medications are the H-2 receptor antagonists, or H-2 blockers, and the proton pump inhibitors. The purpose of these drugs is to decrease the acidity in the stomach and intestinal tract. Less acid frequently improves the symptoms of acid indigestion and decreases the pain when an ulcer is present, but the absorption of numerous vitamins and minerals requires a slightly acidic pH in the intestinal tract. When these drugs make the intestinal tract less acidic, they inhibit the absorption of many nutrients.

Gastritis (inflammation of the cells lining the stomach and/or intestinal tract) and ulcers often are caused by a bacteria known as *Helicobacter pylori,* or *H. pylori.* Actually, *H. pylori* is the most common gastric infection worldwide, and some experts estimate that 90% of ulcers are caused by this bacterium. *H. pylori* causes gastritis and ulcers by burrowing through the protective mucous layer that lines the stomach and intestinal tract.

Taking one of these anti-ulcer drugs decreases the amount of acid, which reduces the pain in the inflamed or ulcerated tissue. *H. pylori,* however, thrive in an alkaline environment. Therefore, taking anti-ulcer drugs treats the symptoms but does not eradicate the cause of the problem. Creating a more alkaline environment actually increases the likelihood that the *H. pylori* bacteria will grow and multiply.

Currently, several protocols are used to treat ulcers and destroy *H. pylori.* These involve taking one or two different antibiotics along with a proton pump inhibitor for 1 to 2 weeks. A different protocol reported a 30% cure rate in people who took 5 grams of vitamin C daily. This included curing the ulcers and completely eradicating the *H. pylori* bacteria. Because ulcers and infection with *H. pylori* are associated with higher rates of gastric cancer, this issue should be taken very seriously.

The fact that the H-2 blocker drugs have been made available without a prescription creates another level of concern. This allows people to use these drugs indiscriminately without any checks and balances from a health care professional. Most people are not aware of the fact that (a) these drugs treat only the symptoms, and (b) altering the acid/base balance actually creates an environment that is more favorable for *H. pylori*.

■ H-2 BLOCKERS

H-2 blockers deplete vitamin B_{12}, vitamin D, calcium, iron, zinc, and folic acid.

Protein is essential to the diet to provide needed amino acids, the building blocks for enzymes that run virtually all body functions. Poor protein absorption can lead to muscle breakdown, weaken the immune system, and result in a host of other problems. H-2 blockers inhibit the body's ability to digest protein.

• **H-2 blockers and vitamin B_{12} depletion:** Stomach acid and pepsin are required to cleave or separate vitamin B_{12} from food, and then a protein known as intrinsic factor is necessary for vitamin B_{12} absorption. All of these processes require a slightly acidic environment. Taking anti-ulcer drugs, which decreases acidity, inhibits vitamin B_{12} digestion and absorption processes. Vitamin B_{12} deficiency can cause anemia, which results in fatigue, tiredness, and weakness, and B_{12} deficiency is also a common cause of depression, especially in elderly people. An inadequate level of B_{12} increases homocysteine, which is a risk factor for cardiovascular disease. If serious B_{12} deficiencies are not corrected, long-term irreversible neurological damage can occur.

• **H-2 blockers and vitamin D depletion:** These drugs seem to inhibit the metabolism of vitamin D, which can lead to osteoporosis and other skeletal problems. Vitamin D is necessary for calcium absorption, which means that insufficient vitamin D could contribute to a calcium deficiency. Vitamin D depletion also can result in muscle weakness and hearing loss.

• **H-2 blockers and calcium depletion:** Studies have been contradictory, so at this time it is not clear if calcium supplements are necessary. The alterations in calcium may be secondary to the effects on vitamin D metabolism. If calcium is truly depleted, it can lead to skeletal problems such as osteoporosis and osteomalacia.

Calcium deficiency also can cause high blood pressure, muscle cramps, heart palpitation, tooth decay, back and leg pains, insomnia, and nervous disorders. It is known, however, that to be optimally absorbed, calcium requires an acidic environment.

• *H-2 blockers and iron depletion:* Iron depletion can cause anemia, which produces weakness and fatigue. Other symptoms associated with iron deficiency include hair loss, brittle nails, and a weakened immune system. Nevertheless, iron supplementation is not recommended unless a lab test determines the presence of iron deficiency.

• *H-2 blockers and zinc depletion:* Zinc is important to a healthy immune system. Zinc is required to produce mature T killer cells in the thymus gland. Deficiencies in zinc result in thymic involution, which results in the development of immature killer cells and reduced immunity. Indications of zinc deficiency are slow healing of wounds and a weakened immune system. Insufficient zinc also can cause insulin resistance, loss of the senses of taste and smell, and infertility and sexual dysfunction in men and women alike.

• *H-2 blockers and folic acid depletion:* Therapy with H-2 blocker drugs causes a slight but noticeable reduction in folic acid levels. Folic acid depletions could become significant during long-term or intensive use of these medications, especially in individuals who are on diets that supply only small amounts of folic acid to begin with. A deficiency of folic acid can cause a wide range of health problems including anemia, depression, cervical dysplasia, birth defects, and increased risks for cardiovascular disease, breast cancer, and colorectal cancer. For a detailed discussion of the problems associated with folic acid deficiency, see pages 50–51.

■ PROTON PUMP INHIBITORS

Proton pump inhibitors deplete vitamin B_{12}. (see the introductory section to Anti-Ulcer Drugs, pages 23.

In 2002, the proton pump inhibitor Prilosec was the number-four-selling drug in the United States, topping $3.5 billion in sales (approximately 1.8% of the market). Prilosec recently was awarded over-the-counter (OTC) status.[16]

Like the H-2 receptor antagonists, the proton pump inhibitors function by decreasing the amount of acidity in the intestinal tract. The difference is that these two classes of anti-ulcer drugs decrease acidity by two different mechanisms, yet the net result is the same — a change in the acid/base levels in the intestinal tract.

To date, studies have reported that the proton pump inhibitors deplete only vitamin B_{12}, whereas the H-2 receptor antagonists deplete vitamin B_{12}, folic acid, vitamin D, calcium, iron, and zinc. One possible explanation for these differences is that the proton pump inhibitors are a much newer class of drugs so studies researching other nutrient depletions have yet to be conducted. It is certainly likely that altered acid/base levels will inhibit the absorption of many nutrients in addition to vitamin B_{12}.

• **Proton pump inhibitors and vitamin B_{12} depletion:** Stomach acid and pepsin are required to cleave or separate vitamin B_{12} from food, and then a protein known as intrinsic factor is necessary for vitamin B_{12} absorption. To proceed, all of these processes require a slightly acidic environment. Taking anti-ulcer drugs, which decreases acidity, inhibits vitamin B_{12} digestion and absorption processes.

A deficiency in Vitamin B_{12} can cause anemia, which results in fatigue, tiredness, and weakness, and a B_{12} deficiency is also a common cause of depression, especially in elderly people. Inadequate levels of B_{12} cause elevated homocysteine, which poses increased risk for cardiovascular disease. If serious B_{12} deficiencies are not corrected, long-term irreversible neurological damage can occur.

MISCELLANEOUS DRUGS

The miscellaneous drugs discussed here are so named because they don't fit the prior categories. Nevertheless, they are prescribed often and have been studied in terms of the nutrients they deplete. The drugs discussed here are methotrexate, penicillamine, EDTA, and ritodrine.

■ METHOTREXATE

Methotrexate depletes folic acid.

• **Methotrexate and folic acid depletion:** Initially, methotrexate was used as a form of cancer chemotherapy. When it is used in cancer therapy, the drug interferes with cancer metabolism by inhibiting the metabolism of folic acid, so folic acid supplementation is not appropriate. Methotrexate, however, is now being used for other conditions such as rheumatoid arthritis. Studies have reported that folic acid supplementation does not reduce the therapeutic effectiveness of methotrexate when it is used for arthritis but it may have a positive effect in lowering the toxic side effects associated with the drug.

A deficiency of folic acid can cause a wide range of health problems including anemia, depression, cervical dysplasia, and birth defects, as well as increased risks for developing cardiovascular disease, breast cancer, and colorectal cancer. For a detailed discussion of the problems associated with folic acid deficiency, see pages 50–51.

■ PENICILLAMINE

Penicillamine is used to treat copper, mercury, zinc, and lead poisoning by promoting the urinary excretion of those metals.

Penicillamine depletes copper, vitamin B_6, magnesium, and zinc.

• **Penicillamine and copper depletion:** Penicillamine therapy causes a substantial increase in urinary copper excretion. Copper depletion can result in anemia and fatigue, problems with the maintenance and repair of connective tissues, and elevated levels of serum cholesterol.

• **Penicillamine and vitamin B_6 depletion:** Vitamin B_6 (pyridoxine) depletion can cause depression and insomnia, as well as increased risk for cardiovascular disease.

   – *Depression:* Vitamin B_6 is necessary for converting the amino acid tryptophan into the neurotransmitter serotonin. A deficiency of serotonin in the brain is strongly associated with depression. Therefore, people taking drugs that deplete vitamin B_6 are at greater risk for depression.

   – *Insomnia:* In the brain, serotonin is converted into melatonin, a hormone that controls sleep. Because a vitamin B_6 deficiency inhibits the synthesis of serotonin, it also will decrease the amount of melatonin that can be produced in the brain. People who become deficient in melatonin will suffer from insomnia and related sleep problems.

   – *Cardiovascular disease:* Vitamin B_6 is one of the B-vitamins that are necessary to metabolize homocysteine, an amino acid produced from the metabolism of the essential amino acid methionine. Homocysteine is a toxic substance capable of directly injuring the lining of the arteries, which is the type of damage that causes atherosclerosis. Under normal conditions, it exists only briefly. A lack of vitamin B_6, however, will produce elevated homocysteine in the blood, and even slight elevations of homocysteine represent a seriously increased risk for developing atherosclerosis, the leading cause of heart disease.

• **Penicillamine and magnesium depletion:** This combination can cause cardiac arrhythmias, high blood pressure, and various other cardiovascular-related problems. Additional conditions associated with low magnesium levels include anxiety, nervousness, insomnia, palpitation, osteoporosis, muscle cramps, muscle weakness, fatigue, PMS, and an increase in the frequency and severity of asthma attacks.

• **Penicillamine and zinc depletion:** The mineral zinc is important to a healthy immune system. Zinc deficiency can cause slow healing of wounds and a weakened immune system. Insufficient zinc also results in insulin resistance, loss of the senses of taste and smell, and infertility and sexual dysfunction in men and women alike.

■ EDTA

EDTA (ethylene-diamine tetraacetic acid) is often given intravenously as chelation therapy. EDTA interacts with calcium, causing excess urinary calcium loss.

EDTA depletes calcium.

• **EDTA and calcium depletion:** Depletion of this mineral can result in skeletal problems such as osteoporosis and osteomalacia. Calcium deficiency also can also cause high blood pressure, muscle cramps, heart palpitation, tooth decay, back and leg pains, insomnia, and nervous disorders.

■ RITODRINE

Ritodrine inhibits uterine contractions. It is used to delay or prevent contractions in women who are going into pre-term labor.

Ritodrine depletes calcium and potassium.

• **Ritodrine and calcium depletion:** Calcium depletion under these conditions will most likely cause symptoms of high blood pressure, muscle cramps, heart palpitation, back and leg pains, insomnia, and nervousness.

• **Ritodrine and potassium depletion:** Potassium depletion can produce symptoms of muscular weakness, tetany (muscle spasms), and postural hypotension (a term that refers to low blood pressure when changing from a lying or sitting position to a standing position), which can cause dizziness and fainting spells. Other symptoms associated with potassium depletion are irregular heartbeat, poor reflexes, fatigue, continuous thirst, edema, constipation, mental confusion, and nervousness.

NOTES

1. "IMS Health," *Pharmacy Times*, April 2002.
2. See Note 1.
3. See Note 1.
4. See Note 1.
5. J. F. Adams, J. S. Clark, et al., "Malabsorption of Vitamin B_{12} and Intrinsic Factor Secretion during Biguanide Therapy," *Diabetologia* (Jan. 1983), Vol. 24, No. 1, pp. 16–18.
6. See Note 1.
7. See Note 1.

8. See Note 1.
9. See Note 1.
10. See Note 1.
11. See Note 1.
12. See Note 1.
13. See Note 1.
14. See Note 1.
15. See Note 1.
16. See Note 1.

To understand the full impact of drug-induced nutrient depletions, we have to understand the importance of each vitamin and mineral to body functioning. This part of the book reviews each of the body nutrients affected by taking the various drugs.

NUTRIENT REVIEWS

PART

III

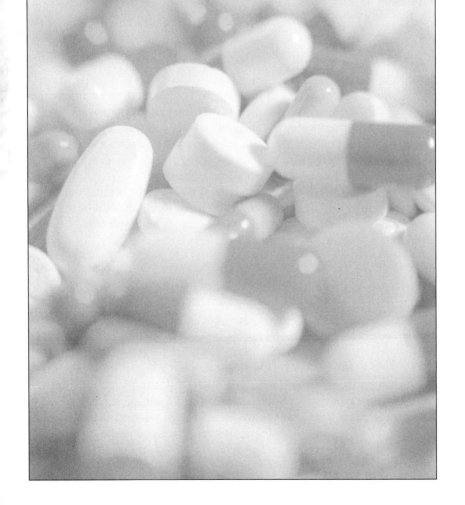

BETA-CAROTENE

Drugs that deplete beta-carotene

- CHOLESTYRAMINE
- COLCHICINE

- COLCHICINE AND
  PROBENICID
- COLESTIPOL

- MINERAL OIL
- NEOMYCIN
- ORLISTAT

BETA-CAROTENE belongs to a group of plant compounds called carotenoids. To date, more than 500 carotenoids have been found in nature. Beta-carotene is the most abundant carotenoid in foods that people eat and is thought to be the most important carotenoid for humans.

Beta-carotene also is known as provitamin A, a precursor of vitamin A in fruits and vegetables. It consists of two molecules of vitamin A linked together. Enzymes in the lining of the intestinal tract split beta-carotene into two separate molecules of vitamin A whenever the body needs it.

■ SYMPTOMS AND CAUSES OF DEFICIENCY

Because beta-carotene is the dietary precursor of vitamin A, deficiencies of this nutrient are the same as deficiencies in vitamin A. Low dietary intake of beta-carotene is associated with a weakened immune system, probably a result of increased damage from free radicals. Many types of cancer, including epithelial cell cancers, are associated with low dietary intake of beta-carotene. Additional effects are dry, scaly and rough skin; xeropthalmia (night blindness); and bone deformities.

Several drugs are capable of reducing blood levels of beta-carotene. The main cause of a deficiency, however, is not eating enough of the colored fruits and vegetables that are known to contain ample beta-carotene.

■ BIOLOGICAL FUNCTIONS AND EFFECTS

Beta-carotene functions as a chain-breaking antioxidant. This means that it traps free radicals, which stops the chain reaction of free radical destruction. Beta-carotene is the natural agent that is most capable of quenching singlet oxygen free radicals in humans.

■ SIDE EFFECTS AND TOXICITY

No known toxicities are associated with beta-carotene. Ingesting large doses of beta-carotene, however, can result in a harmless side effect called carotenosis. This orange coloration is most noticeable on the palms of the hands and the soles of the feet. The discoloration subsides when the dosage is lowered or stopped.

■ RDA and Dosage

No RDA has been established for beta-carotene. The most common supplemental dose of beta-carotene is 10,000 I.U. daily.

■ Food Sources

Beta-carotene occurs exclusively in plant (fruit and vegetable) foods. Foods containing high amounts of beta-carotene include:

- green leafy vegetables
- carrots
- squash
- apricots
- cantaloupe
- sweet potatoes
- spinach
- peaches
- green, yellow, and red peppers

BIFIDOBACTERIA BIFIDUM (BIFIDUS)

Drugs that deplete bifidobacteria bifidum

- ■ Aminoglycosides
- ■ Cephalosporins
- ■ Chemotherapeutics
- ■ Co-trimoxazole
- ■ Fluoroquinolones
- ■ Macrolides
- ■ Penicillins
- ■ Sulfonamides
- ■ Tetracyclines

BIFIDOBACTERIA BIFIDUM, also known as bifidus, is the main strain of beneficial bacteria that inhabit the large intestine. If the balance between the beneficial and the pathological bacteria gets upset, a condition known as dysbiosis develops. A frequent cause of dysbiosis is the use of antibiotics. When a person takes antibiotics, most of the bifidobacteria are killed along with the pathological bacteria. Healthy colonizations of intestinal microflora with beneficial bacteria such as *L. acidophilus* and *Acidophilus bifidus* are key to maintaining a healthy immune system. Products containing beneficial bacteria are frequently referred to as probiotics.

■ Symptoms and Causes of Deficiency

Symptoms of a deficiency of bifidobacteria bifidum include gas, bloating, diarrhea or constipation, and bad breath.

The primary cause of a deficiency is the use of antibiotic drugs. Other causes include prolonged high stress levels, exposure to or ingestion of toxic metals or pesticides, and a poor diet containing large quantities of sugar, fat, and refined and processed foods lacking in fiber content.

■ Biological Functions and Effects

Bifidobacteria produce fatty acids in the colon. This slightly increases the acidic environment, making it unfavorable for the growth of pathological bacteria, yeasts, and molds.

The fatty acids that the bifidobacteria produce are the main source of energy for the colonocytes, the cells that form the inner surface of the colon.

■ SIDE EFFECTS AND TOXICITY

No toxicity is associated with probiotics, and they do not interfere with other medications.

■ RDA AND DOSAGE

No RDA has been set. Dosages for probiotics are measured in cfu's (colony forming units), which refers to the number of viable (live) organisms. Many probiotic products contain a combination of acidophilus and bifidobacteria.

To prevent problems, healthy people can take a probiotic containing 1–2 billion cfu per day. Individuals with dysbiosis and those who are taking antibiotics should take 10–15 billion cfu (a combination of acidophilus and bifidobacteria) twice daily for 2 weeks.

■ FOOD SOURCES

Because foods do not contain substantial amounts of bifidobacteria, they are best obtained by purchasing commercial probiotic products containing bifidobacteria.

BIOTIN

Drugs that deplete biotin

■ AMIONGLYCOSIDES	■ MACROLIDES	■ PRIMIDONE
■ BARBITURATES	■ PENICILLINS	■ SULFONAMIDES
■ CARBAMAZEPINE	■ PHENOBARBITAL	■ TETRACYCLINES
■ CEPHALOSPORINS	■ PHENYTOIN	■ TRIMETHOPRIM
■ FLUOROQUINOLONES		

BIOTIN is one of the more recently discovered water-soluble B vitamins. It was first isolated in 1936 and was synthesized in 1943. Biotin is essential to many enzyme systems. Biotin consumed from plant and animal sources is bound to proteins, and the biotin is not released until it comes in contact with the enzymes in the upper part of the small intestine. It also is absorbed from the lower part of the small intestine, where it is synthesized by the "friendly" intestinal bacteria.

■ SYMPTOMS AND CAUSES OF DEFICIENCY

Biotin deficiency in humans is rare. Some diabetic individuals have an abnormality in a biotin-dependent enzyme, which can lead to dysfunctions of the nervous system.

Deficiency symptoms include progressive hair loss, loss of hair color, depression, scaly dermatitis, sores on the nose and in the mouth, anorexia, nausea, numbness and tingling of the extremities, muscle pain, and heart irregularities.

■ BIOLOGICAL FUNCTIONS AND EFFECTS

Biotin-containing enzymes play a vital role in the production of energy from the metabolism of carbohydrates and fats. Biotin-containing enzymes also are involved in the manufacture of fats and the excretion of byproducts from the metabolism of protein.

Enzymes containing biotin participate in carboxylation reactions (adding carbon dioxide to acceptor molecules) decarboxylation reactions (which remove carbon dioxide) and deamination reactions (removing NH_2 groups from certain amino acids).

Biotin is the vitamin that produces healthy hair and helps to prevent graying and baldness. Supplementation in cases of severe deficiency will help, but because biotin deficiency is rare, these claims are suspect. Biotin does help with "uncombable hair syndrome," a condition in which children have multiple cowlicks (the hair sticks up in all directions and won't lie down). In many cases, biotin helps people with dry, splitting fingernails.

■ SIDE EFFECTS AND TOXICITY

Biotin has no known toxic effects. Excessive levels are easily eliminated through urination.

■ RDA AND DOSAGE

The RDA for biotin is 0.3 milligrams (mg) per day. Pharmacologic doses in the scientific literature range from 0.3 mg up to 3 mg. Because biotin is rarely deficient in humans, taking large doses is seldom necessary.

■ FOOD SOURCES

Biotin is found abundantly in many plant and animal foods. A considerable amount of biotin also is synthesized by the "friendly" intestinal bacteria. The best food sources are:

- liver
- milk
- brewer's yeast
- bananas
- grapefruit
- watermelon
- strawberries
- peanuts

Drugs that deplete boron

NO STUDIES REPORTING DRUG-INDUCED BORON DEPLETION HAVE BEEN FOUND.

BORON is a trace mineral that is most prevalent in nature as borax, a mixture of boron, sodium, and oxygen. Although boron has been recognized as an essential nutrient for plants for more than a century, not until the mid-1980s was it discovered to be essential to humans. Therefore, some of the information about its metabolic activity and function is still speculative. Research during the past decade has strongly implicated that boron plays vital roles in metabolism and the health of bones.

■ SYMPTOMS AND CAUSES OF DEFICIENCY

A deficiency of boron results in increased loss of calcium and magnesium through the urine. This leads to more rapid bone demineralization, which probably hastens the development of osteoporosis in post-menopausal women.

■ BIOLOGICAL FUNCTIONS AND EFFECTS

Boron has several important effects:

1. Boron influences the metabolism of calcium and therefore may play a role in preventing osteoporosis in postmenopausal women, as boron has been shown to substantially reduce calcium loss through the urine. In one study, when boron was given to women deficient in boron, it produced a 44% reduction in the urinary excretion of calcium.[1]

2. Relatedly, boron may influence the synthesis of vitamin D, which plays a role in preventing bone loss, and in the metabolism of magnesium.

3. Boron has a regulatory effect on the production of estrogens and testosterone. Biochemically, boron facilitates hydroxylation reactions. Because the synthesis of estrogens and testosterone both require hydroxylation, there is strong indication that boron influences production of these hormones.

People living in geographical areas with low levels of boron in the soil have a higher than usual incidence of osteoarthritis.

■ SIDE EFFECTS AND TOXICITY

An excessive intake of boron can cause nausea, vomiting, diarrhea, skin rashes, and fatigue. No health or medical problems have been reported in areas of the world where the daily diet supplies up to 41 mg per day of boron.

■ RDA AND DOSAGE

No RDA has been set for boron. Based on animal studies, the human requirement for boron is estimated to be from 1 to 2 mg/day. Pharmacological doses in the scientific literature range from 3 mg to 6 gm daily.

Available forms of boron are sodium borate and boron chelates, the latter of which include boron citrate, aspartate, and glycinate.

■ FOOD SOURCES

Boron is readily available from fruits and vegetables, and it is easily absorbed from the intestinal tract.

CALCIUM

Drugs that deplete calcium

■ ALUMINUM HYDROXIDE-CONTAINING PRODUCTS	■ CYCLOSERINE	■ MAGNESIUM-CONTAINING PRODUCTS
■ AMINOGLYCOSIDES	■ DIGOXIN	■ MINERAL OIL
■ AMPHOTERICIN B	■ EDTA	■ NIZATIDINE
■ ASPIRIN	■ ETHACRYNIC ACID	■ PHENOBARTIBAL
■ BARBITURATES	■ ESTROGEN	■ PHENYTOIN
■ BUMETANIDE	■ FAMOTIDINE	■ RANITIDINE
■ CARBAMAZEPINE	■ FOSPHENYTOIN	■ SUCRALFATE
■ CHOLESTYRAMINE	■ FUROSEMIDE	■ TETRACYCLINES
■ CIMETIDINE	■ HYDROCHOLOR-THIAZIDE AND TRIAMTERENE	■ TORSEMIDE
■ COLCHICINE		■ TRIAMTERENE
■ CORTICOSTEROIDS		■ ZONISAMIDE

CALCIUM is the most abundant mineral in the human body, and the fifth most common substance behind carbon, hydrogen, oxygen, and nitrogen. Average healthy male bodies contain about 2.5 to 3 pounds of calcium, and female bodies contain about 2 pounds. Approximately 99% of the body calcium is present in the bones and teeth, which leaves only about 1% in cells and body fluids. Even though only a small amount of calcium is in the blood, the body goes to great lengths to maintain blood-calcium levels within a relatively narrow range.

Three regulatory mechanisms control blood-calcium. If levels drop too low:

1. The intestines absorb calcium at a faster rate.

2. The bones release more calcium.

3. The kidneys excrete less calcium.

In addition, phosphorus displaces calcium. Eating a lot of foods that contain phosphorus promotes increased urinary excretion of calcium, which in turn can prompt the body to leach calcium from the bones and thereby contribute to osteoporosis. The main sources of dietary phosphorus are soft drinks and animal protein.

Calcium exists in bones and teeth primarily as hydroxyapatite, a calcium carbonate/calcium phosphate compound that gives these tissues rigidity and strength.

■ SYMPTOMS AND CAUSES OF DEFICIENCY

Rickets is the classic calcium-deficiency disease. It occurs most frequently in children and results in a variety of bone deformities. A lack of vitamin D and of sunshine (which promotes the formation of Vitamin D in the body) can produce the calcium deficiency that leads to rickets. The two most prevalent adult conditions caused by calcium deficiency are osteoporosis and osteomalacia, characterized by bone deformities and a propensity for fractures.

Symptoms of calcium deficiency include muscle cramps, heart palpitation, high blood pressure, brittle or soft bones, tooth decay, back and leg pains, insomnia, and nervous disorders.

The following are additional causes of calcium deficiency:

• Magnesium deficiency causes various abnormalities in the metabolism of calcium.

• Eating foods that are high in phosphorus (soft drinks and animal protein) promotes the urinary loss of calcium.

• Inflammatory conditions in the intestinal tract decrease the body's absorption of calcium.

Other significant factors that can lower calcium levels include caffeine intake, excess dietary fat and fiber, lack of exercise, and the numerous drugs that can cause calcium depletion.

■ BIOLOGICAL FUNCTIONS AND EFFECTS

The most important documented function of calcium is its role in the development and maintenance of healthy bones and teeth. The needs for calcium are greatest in childhood and adolescence, and during pregnancy and lactation.

Additional functions of calcium in the body are the following:

• Calcium helps to initiate muscle contractions. As such, it plays a vital role in the contraction–relaxation cycle that regulates normal heartbeat.

• Calcium is involved in several steps of the blood-clotting mechanism.

- Ionized calcium regulates the passage of fluids across cellular membranes by affecting the permeability of cell walls.
- Calcium activates various enzyme systems responsible for muscle contraction, fat digestion, and protein metabolism.

Calcium supplements are only minimally effective when they are taken alone. In one study of osteoporosis, a nutritional supplement containing a broad range of micronutrients, bone density increased two to three times more effectively than calcium alone.[2]

Low levels of calcium are associated with hypertension, and many studies have shown that the blood pressure of hypertensive patients who take calcium supplements is slightly lowered. The gains are so small, though, that calcium supplements cannot be suggested as a treatment.

Several studies report that men with low levels of calcium intake have higher rates of colorectal cancer. Calcium supplementation in high-risk individuals decreases the rate of abnormal cell division in the colon.

■ SIDE EFFECTS AND TOXICITY

The body efficiently excretes calcium, so large doses usually do not produce toxic effects. Taking large doses of calcium regularly, however, may interfere with the absorption of zinc, iron, and magnesium.

■ RDA AND DOSAGE

The RDA for calcium is 1000 mg/day. Pharmacologic doses in the scientific literature range from 1000 mg to 2000 mg/day.

Available forms are calcium citrate, aspartate, ascorbate, lactate, phosphate, carbonate, glycinate, malate, amino acid chelates, and microcrystalline hydroxyapatite compound (MCHC).

■ FOOD SOURCES

The major sources of dietary calcium for most people are milk and dairy products. The appropriateness of cow's milk as a source of calcium has been questioned because (1) milk is a frequent cause of food allergies; (2) many people have digestive problems as a result of lactose intolerance; (3) an enzyme from cow's milk, xanthine oxidase, can damage the arterial membranes, and antibodies to bovine (cow) xanthine oxidase have been found in the blood of individuals who have atherosclerosis.

Other good food sources are dark green leafy vegetables, broccoli, legumes, nuts, and whole grains.

CARNITINE

ALTHOUGH CARNITINE is a nonessential amino acid, it has vitamin-like properties. It can be synthesized from the essential amino acids lysine and methionine. The highest concentrations of carnitine are found in the heart, muscles, liver, and kidney.

■ SYMPTOMS AND CAUSES OF DEFICIENCY

Carnitine deficiencies are rare because the body produces carnitine relatively easily. Effects of deficiency include elevated levels of blood lipids, abnormal liver function, and impaired glucose control. Symptoms are muscle weakness and lowered energy level.

■ BIOLOGICAL FUNCTIONS AND EFFECTS

The primary function of carnitine seems to be the regulation of heart function by controlling the production of energy in muscle tissue. Additional functions are the following.

• Carnitine regulates fat metabolism by facilitating the transport of fats across cell membranes into the mitochondria for energy production.

• Carnitine helps the body oxidize amino acids to produce energy when necessary.

• Carnitine helps to metabolize ketones.

• Although this use has not been well researched, many athletes take carnitine supplements to increase their energy and endurance.

• The ability of carnitine to increase the oxidation of fats suggests that it might be useful in weight-loss diets.

■ SIDE EFFECTS AND TOXICITY

Carnitine seems to be safe, with no significant side effects reported, even at high doses.

■ RDA AND DOSAGE

No RDA has been established for carnitine. The dosage range for carnitine is 1500–4000 mg/day in divided doses.

■ FOOD SOURCES

Animal food sources include, meat, poultry, and dairy products.

CHLORIDE

Drugs that deplete chloride

NO STUDIES REPORTING DRUG-INDUCED DEPLETION OF CHLORIDE HAVE BEEN FOUND.

CHLORIDE is one of the body's three major electrolytes, the other two being sodium and potassium. Electrolytes are the dissociated ions, responsible for osmotic pressure in body fluids. Osmotic pressure is rigidly controlled, primarily by regulatory mechanisms that determine the rate of resorption of ions and water through the kidneys. The ionic strength of electrolytes enables them to influence the solubility of proteins and other substances throughout the body.

Control of chloride, sodium, and potassium is mediated by the hormones of the adrenal cortex and the anterior pituitary gland. Chloride and the other electrolytes are readily absorbed through the intestinal tract and are excreted primarily in the urine and sweat. Under normal conditions, chloride represents about 3% of the total mineral content of the body.

■ SYMPTOMS AND CAUSES OF DEFICIENCY

Chloride deficiency is rare because of the widespread availability and use of salt (sodium chloride). A deficiency creates a condition called metabolic alkalosis, which can cause diarrhea, vomiting and sweating. Other symptoms of chloride deficiency include weakness, poor digestion, loss of appetite, and hair loss.

A deficiency in chloride can be caused by extensive diarrhea, frequent vomiting, adrenal insufficiency, long-term use of diuretics, and systemic acidosis. Profuse sweating also can cause chloride depletion.

■ BIOLOGICAL FUNCTIONS AND EFFECTS

Chloride is the primary anion functioning in the extracellular fluids throughout the body, which include the blood, lymph, and the fluid in the spaces between cells. Approximately 85% of the chloride ions reside in extracellular fluids and 15% in the intracellular fluids.

Additional effects include the following.

• Chloride, along with sodium and potassium, helps to maintain normal osmotic equilibrium by controlling the distribution and balance of water throughout the body.

- Along with phosphate and sulfate ions, chloride helps to maintain the acid/alkaline pH balance throughout the body.

- As part of the hydrochloric acid in the stomach, chloride is necessary to maintain the normal acidity of the stomach for the processes of digestion.

- Chloride helps regulate removal of CO_2 (carbon dioxide) from cells and its transport to the lungs for excretion.

- Chloride and the other electrolytes, in conjunction with calcium and magnesium, maintain transmission of nerve impulses and normal muscle activity (contraction and relaxation).

■ SIDE EFFECTS AND TOXICITY

Excess chloride is efficiently excreted through the kidneys and, therefore, chloride toxicity is virtually impossible in humans. Because of the efficient excretion of excess chloride, side effects are not an issue.

■ RDA AND DOSAGE

No RDA has been set for chloride because it is so readily available in foods. Estimated safe and adequate intake of chloride for adults is from 1.5 to 5 grams/day.

■ FOOD SOURCES

The primary dietary source of chloride is table salt (sodium chloride). Chloride also occurs abundantly in vegetables and animal foods.

CHOLINE

Drugs that deplete choline

NO STUDIES THAT REPORT CHOLINE DEPLETION HAVE BEEN FOUND.

CHOLINE is a member of the water-soluble B vitamin group. Classifying choline as a vitamin is questionable because the human body synthesizes it naturally. Because the rate of synthesis is not normally sufficient to meet human metabolic needs, however, choline has been included as an essential vitamin nutrient.

■ SYMPTOMS AND CAUSES OF DEFICIENCY

A deficiency of choline in humans is virtually nonexistent.

■ BIOLOGICAL FUNCTIONS AND EFFECTS

Choline is the precursor to, and a component of, the neurotransmitter acetylcholine. As such, choline is intimately involved in a wide range of neurological activities, including the functions of movement, coordination, and the stimulation of muscle contraction. It also plays a vital role in the brain functions of thought, memory, and intellect.

Specific functions of choline are the following.

• Choline is a lipotropic (fat-emulsifying) agent.

• Structurally, choline contains three methyl groups that enable it to serve as a methyl donor in many important biochemical pathways.

• Choline is a part of phosphatidyl choline, a phospholipid that is a major structural component of cell walls and cellular membranes throughout the body, functioning in the metabolism of fat and in the transport of fat from the liver.

• After being converted to betaine, choline functions in the synthesis of amino acids and proteins.

One of the main characteristics of Alzheimer's disease is a deficiency of acetylcholine. With high doses of phosphatidyl choline, some individuals with mild to moderate Alzheimer's disease show improved memory and cognitive function.

Choline is useful in reducing the tremors associated with tardive dyskinesia and other diseases of the nervous system.

■ SIDE EFFECTS AND TOXICITY

The toxicity of choline is very low.

Side effects of orally taking high doses of choline salts such as choline chloride can readily produce nausea, diarrhea, and dizziness.

Taking choline orally produces an unpleasant "fishy" odor as a result of intestinal bacteria metabolizing the choline and releasing the odorous substance trimethylamine.

■ RDA AND DOSAGE

No RDA has been set for choline.

Pharmacologic doses in the scientific literature range from 2 grams up to 10 grams in divided doses. Larger doses are not recommended because they cause diarrhea and the unpleasant "fishy" odor.

Available forms are choline bitartrate, choline citrate, choline chloride, CDP-choline, and as a component of phosphatidyl choline, also known as lecithin.

■ FOOD SOURCES

The richest source of dietary choline is egg yolk. Other good sources are organ meats, brewer's yeast, wheat germ, soy beans, peanuts and other legumes.

CHROMIUM

CHROMIUM is an essential trace mineral that is commonly deficient in American diets. One survey reported that the diets of 90% of Americans contained less than the Recommended Dietary Allowance (RDA) for chromium.[3]

Even though the body of an average healthy individual contains only a few milligrams, this small amount plays important roles in enhancing the effectiveness of insulin, regulating blood sugar levels, and activating various enzymes for energy production.

Chromium is biologically active only when it forms complexes with organic compounds. One such complex is the glucose tolerance factor (GTF). In addition to potentiating the effect of insulin, GTF seems to help lower elevated blood cholesterol and triglyceride levels.

■ SYMPTOMS AND CAUSES OF DEFICIENCY

A deficiency of chromium is claimed to be one of the major nutritional insufficiencies in the United States. The main cause of chromium deficiency is low dietary intake. And high sugar consumption is a major contributing cause of chromium deficiency because sugar raises blood chromium levels, which increases urinary excretion and thereby accelerates chromium deficiency.

One of the main indications of chromium deficiency is adult-onset (Type II) diabetes. The deficiency impairs GTF activity, which increases insulin levels. Elevated insulin causes increased urinary excretion of chromium, which makes the deficiency worse, contributing to the development of diabetes. In addition:

- A low level of chromium is associated with cardiovascular disease.

- Disturbances in protein and lipid metabolism have been reported in conjunction with chromium deficiency.

Symptoms of chromium deficiency may parallel those of diabetes, including numbness and tingling in the extremities, neuropathy in the arms and legs, weight gain, erratic energy levels, fatigue, anxiousness, nervousness, and fatigue and headaches when meals are not eaten regularly and frequently.

■ BIOLOGICAL FUNCTIONS AND EFFECTS

Some studies suggest that chromium is helpful in preventing adult-onset (Type II) diabetes. This seems to be a significant finding for a large percentage of the elderly population.

- Chromium, as a component of glucose tolerance, enhances the blood-sugar lowering effects of insulin by facilitating the uptake of glucose into cells. Chromium actually increases the activity of insulin, thereby reducing the amount of insulin required to control blood sugar.

- Many studies indicate that chromium decreases total cholesterol, LDL cholesterol (the "bad" cholesterol), and triglycerides while increasing levels of HDL cholesterol (the "good" cholesterol). Other studies, however, have not shown these benefits.

- In combination with niacin, chromium has been shown to effectively lower elevated blood cholesterol levels. This enables the dose of niacin to be low enough so that niacin flush is no longer a problem. Niacin flush is a vasodilation reaction resulting in redness of the skin and itching, which typically occurs if dosages are in excess of 50 mg at a time

- Chromium may be helpful in the treatment of hypoglycemia.

- Some studies have shown that supplemental chromium increases lean body mass, which enhances body composition. Other studies, however, have shown no improvement in lean body mass.

■ SIDE EFFECTS AND TOXICITY

Side effects and toxicity from taking supplemental chromium are virtually nonexistent in humans.

■ RDA AND DOSAGE

There is no RDA for chromium. In 1989, however, the National Research Council recommended the Safe and Adequate Range for adults to be from 50 to 200 mcg/day. Pharmacologic doses in the scientific literature are frequently in the range of 200 to 400 mcg/day.

Available forms are chromium picolinate, chromium polynicotinate, chromium chloride, and chromium-enriched yeast (yeast grown in a growth medium enriched with chromium).

■ FOOD SOURCES

Good food sources of chromium are:

- whole-grain breads and cereals
- lean meats
- cheese
- black pepper
- thyme

Drugs that deplete coenzyme Q$_{10}$

- ACEBUTOLOL
- ACETOHEXAMIDE
- ADVICOR
- AMITRIPTYLINE
- AMILORIDE
- AMOXAPINE
- ATORVASTATIN
- BENZTHIAZIDE
- BETA-BLOCKERS (INCLUDING PROPRANOLOL, ATENOLOL, AND METOPROLOL, AMONG OTHERS)
- CERIVASTATIN
- CHLOROTHIAZIDE
- CHLORPROMAZINE
- CLOMIPRAMINE
- CLONIDINE
- DESIPRAMINE
- DOXEPIN
- ENOXACIN
- FENOFIBRATE
- FLUPHENAZINE
- FLUVASTATIN
- GEMFIBROZIL
- GLIMEPIRIDE
- GLYBURIDE
- HALOPERIDOL
- HYDRALAZINE
- HYDRALAZINE AND HYDROCHLOROTH-IAZIDE
- HYDRALAZINE, HYDROCHLOROTHIAZIDE, AND RESERPINE
- HYDROCHLORO-THIAZIDE
- HYDROFLUMETHIAZIDE
- IMIPRAMINE
- INDAPAMIDE
- LOVASTATIN
- MESORIDAZINE
- METFORMIN
- METHYCLOTHIAZIDE
- METHYLDOPA
- METOLAZONE
- NORTRIPTYLINE
- PERPHENAZINE
- POLYTHIAZIDE
- PRAVASTATIN
- PROCHLORPERAZINE
- PROMAZINE
- PROMETHAZINE
- PROTRIPTYLINE
- QUINETHAZONE
- SIMVASTATIN
- THIETHYLPERAZINE
- THIORIDAZINE
- TOLAZAMIDE
- TOLBUTAMIDE
- TRICHLOMETHIAZIDE
- TRIFLUOPERAZINE
- TRIMIPRAMINE

COENZYME Q$_{10}$ (CoQ$_{10}$) is one of the most important nutrients in the human body. It is a fat-soluble, vitamin-like compound also known as ubiquinone, from the word ubiquitous, which means "everywhere." Coenzyme Q, or ubiquinone compounds, are synthesized in the cells of all living organisms — plants, animals, and humans. Of the ten coenzyme Q compounds that occur throughout nature, only coenzyme Q$_{10}$ is synthesized in humans.

In 1958, Professor Karl Folkers, while employed at Merck, elucidated the chemical structure of coenzyme Q$_{10}$. Working with tiny quantities, Folkers was able to determine that CoQ$_{10}$ had great promise in treating cardiovascular disease. He was not able to convince his superiors to pursue the development of CoQ$_{10}$, however, because Merck had recently launched its new blockbuster drug in the cardiovascular arena, called Diuril. Consequently, the formula and patent rights for coenzyme Q$_{10}$ were sold to a Japanese company.

The Japanese quickly developed new methods of synthesizing large quantities of coenzyme Q$_{10}$, and it has become one of the best-selling and most effective treatments for cardiovascular disease in Japan.

The benefits of this miracle nutrient, coenzyme Q_{10}, are just beginning to be recognized in the United States.

■ Symptoms and Causes of Deficiency

Dietary sources contain only a limited amount of coenzyme Q_{10}. Most of the CoQ_{10} in humans is manufactured by the body's cells. The biosynthesis of coenzyme Q_{10} is a 17-step process that requires the following nutrients: riboflavin (B_2), niacin (B_3), pantothenic acid (B_5), pyridoxine (B_6), cobalamin (B_{12}), folic acid, vitamin C, and many other trace elements. Consequently, the complex synthesis of coenzyme Q_{10} can be interrupted in many ways. Many people with health problems probably have a deficiency of coenzyme Q_{10} as a result of inadequate dietary intake of the necessary nutrients or ingestion of one or more drugs that interrupt the synthesis of coenzyme Q_{10}.

A deficiency of coenzyme Q_{10} can cause high blood pressure, angina, mitral valve prolapse, stroke, cardiac arrhythmias, cardiomyopathies, congestive heart failure, poor insulin production, lack of energy, gingivitis, and generalized weakening of the immune system.

Coenzyme Q_{10} is intimately involved in the production of energy. Therefore, a deficiency of CoQ_{10} first affects the heart and cardiovascular system because the heart is the most energy-demanding muscle in the human body. The results of some studies suggest that congestive heart failure is primarily a coenzyme Q_{10}-deficiency disease.

■ Biological Functions and Effects

Coenzyme Q_{10} plays essential roles in the production of energy within the mitochondria. It is a coenzyme for numerous enzymes that are involved in the production of adenosine triphosphate (ATP), the high-energy fuel for all living cells.

The following are some effects of coenzyme Q_{10} in the body:

- CoQ_{10} is an important antioxidant. Because it is fat-soluble, it is able to reside in the cell membranes, where it provides protection against damage from free radicals.

- CoQ_{10} is transported in the bloodstream on molecules of LDL-cholesterol. As such, it plays a major role in preventing the oxidation of LDL and reducing the risk of atherosclerosis.

- CoQ_{10} helps to protect against the potential side effects of widely used drugs such as adriamycin, beta-blockers, diuretics, and drugs used for psychiatric disorders.

Administration of the drug is reportedly useful in treating all kinds of cardiovascular diseases, and it has been found to be effective in treating periodontal (gum) disease.

■ SYMPTOMS OF TOXICITY

Coenzyme Q_{10} seems to be safe. No studies have reported toxicity or adverse side effects.

■ RDA AND DOSAGE

No RDA has been set for coenzyme Q_{10}. Normal supplement dosages range from 30 mg to 100 mg per day.

Some reports have indicated treating health conditions such as severe cardiovascular disease and advanced breast cancer with dosages from 300 mg to 360 mg per day. Utilizing high dosages to treat severe health problems should be done only under the supervision of a physician.[4]

■ FOOD SOURCES

Coenzyme Q compounds exist in the cells of all plants and animals. The level of coenzyme Q_{10} that we obtain from the diet, however, is believed to be inadequate to meet our needs for optimal health and wellness. Therefore, supplementation is advisable.

COPPER

Drugs that deplete Copper

■ ABACAVIR	■ STAVUDINE	■ PENICILLAMINE
■ CLOFIBRATE	■ ETHAMBUTOL	■ VALPROIC ACID
■ DIDANOSINE	■ FENOFIBRATE	■ ZALCITABINE
■ DELAVIRDINE	■ NEVIRAPINE	■ ZIDOVUDINE
■ LAMIVUDINE		

COPPER is an essential trace mineral that is a co-factor in many copper-dependent enzyme systems throughout the body. Copper is absorbed in the small intestine and carried to the liver, where it is incorporated into liver enzymes and secreted into the blood on ceruloplasmin. The results of some dietary surveys suggest that the diet of most Americans provides only half of the Recommended Dietary Allowance for copper.

■ SYMPTOMS AND CAUSES OF DEFICIENCY

Although severe copper deficiency is rare, marginal copper deficiency is common, as the diet of many Americans supplies only about 50% of the RDA. A high intake of zinc supplements can lead to copper deficiency because zinc interferes with copper absorption.

Symptoms of copper deficiency include loss of color in the hair and skin (because of decreased synthesis of melanin), anemia, fatigue, low body temperature, breakdown of connective tissue, various cardiovascular problems, nervous system disorders, and reduced resistance to infection.

Some researchers have shown that copper deficiency is associated with elevated blood cholesterol and triglyceride levels, as well as the development of atherosclerosis. Thus, copper deficiency may play a role in the risk of cardiovascular disease.

Menkes' disease, also called kinky or steely hair syndrome, is a genetic defect in copper absorption characterized by stunted growth, abnormalities in cardiovascular and skeletal development, progressive cognitive decline, and premature death.

■ BIOLOGICAL FUNCTIONS AND EFFECTS

Copper is required for the synthesis and function of hemoglobin and, as such, it plays a central role in the transport of oxygen throughout the body. Copper also stimulates the absorption of iron. In addition:

• Copper is required for the synthesis of collagen, which determines the integrity of bone, cartilage, skin, and tendons.

• Copper is involved in the production of elastin.

• Copper is required for the production of melanin, which imparts color to the skin and hair, Copper is a component of many important enzymes.

Because copper chelates are anti-inflammatory agents, they are effective in combating some forms of arthritis. A double-blind study has shown that wearing copper bracelets helps some arthritic individuals.[5]

The role of copper in cardiovascular disease remains controversial. Various studies have shown that both high and low copper levels can increase cardiovascular abnormalities.

Some studies have indicated that copper may play a role in osteoporosis and diabetes.

■ SIDE EFFECTS AND TOXICITY

Copper toxicity is rare, occurring only when intakes are about 200 to 500 times above normal. Side effects include intestinal disturbances, excess production of saliva, a metallic taste in the mouth, headache, dizziness, and weakness. Severe cases cause hypertension, liver damage, kidney failure, and possibly even death.

In cases of elevated copper, the problems that develop may not be a result of copper toxicity but, rather, its interference with the absorption and distribution of other metal ions such as iron and zinc.

Wilson's disease is a genetic disorder that causes a toxic accumulation of copper in the liver, kidney, cornea of the eye, and central nervous system. Treatment involves a low-copper diet and use of penicillamine, which facilitates the excretion of copper.

Occasional copper toxicity has been reported in individuals who live in houses with copper water pipes that leach copper into the drinking water.

■ RDA AND DOSAGE

The RDA for copper is 2 mg per day. Pharmacologic doses of copper in scientific studies usually range from 2 mg to 4 mg/day.

Available forms are copper gluconate, amino acid chelates, glycinate, lysinate, citrate, sulfate, and sebacate.

■ FOOD SOURCES

Copper-containing foods include:

- organ meats
- whole-grain breads and cereals
- shellfish, including oysters
- dark green leafy vegetables
- dried legumes
- nuts
- chocolate

FLUORIDE

Drugs that deplete fluoride

NO STUDIES REPORTING DRUG-INDUCED FLUORIDE DEPLETIONS HAVE BEEN FOUND.

FLUORIDE is a controversial nutrient, and fluoridation of community water supplies is the main issue. Proponents claim that fluoridation reduces the incidence of dental caries (cavities) and strengthens the bones. Opponents claim that fluoridation does more harm than good. This issue is far from being resolved. Hotly contested, emotionally charged debates are taking place in scientific journals and in communities that are considering fluoridation.

It is generally accepted that fluoride prevents cavities and has an effect on bone metabolism. Fluoride hardens tooth enamel and increases the stability of the bone mineral matrix. As a result, teeth are less prone to developing cavities and bones are less susceptible to osteoporosis.

Critics of fluoridation of water supplies, however, cite studies indicating that children in cities with fluoridated water have about the same incidence of dental caries as those in communities with nonfluoridated water supplies. Critics also cite studies reporting higher rates of bone fractures in fluoridated communities.

Cancer is another concern. In 1977, results of a study presented at a Congressional hearing revealed that people living in the ten largest fluoridated U.S. cities had a 10% higher incidence of cancer than those living in the ten largest non-fluoridated cities.[6] In 1989, the American Dental Association reduced its longstanding official estimate of 60% benefit and stated that fluoride provides a 25% reduction in tooth decay. In 2003 the American Dental Association states that the tooth decay is occurring at pre-fluoridation rates, and the association attributes this to the high consumption of soda pop.

Whether municipal water supplies should or should not be fluoridated is a medical, social, and political issue that is far from being resolved. Two points in the fluoride debate are beyond argument.

1. Ingesting too much fluoride can produce a number of undesirable side effects.

2. The dosage range between benefits and undesirable side effects is relatively narrow, and sensitivity to fluoride varies widely from person to person.

■ SYMPTOMS AND CAUSES OF DEFICIENCY

The major symptom of fluoride deficiency is an increase in the incidence of dental caries in areas of the country where natural levels of fluoride are low and municipal water supplies are not fluoridated.

■ BIOLOGICAL FUNCTIONS AND EFFECTS

The primary function of fluoride is to prevent dental caries. In children, fluoride creates stronger teeth because it gets incorporated into dental structure when the teeth are being formed. Therefore, the effects of fluoride are greatest when it is ingested during early childhood when teeth are still forming. After teeth have erupted, topical fluoride is deposited into the enamel, creating a stronger protective surface.

Fluoride replaces the hydroxy portion of hydroxyapatite in bones, producing a less water-soluble, more stable substance called fluorapatite.

Some reports suggest that fluoride protects against osteoporosis and also is useful in treating osteoporosis. Fluoride works in conjunction with calcium to stimulate new bone growth, and it also is incorporated into the bone, making the bones stronger. Some dissenting studies, however, report that fluoride makes bones more brittle and prone to fracture.

■ SIDE EFFECTS AND TOXICITY

The main side effect from excess fluoride is fluorosis, a mottling discoloration of the teeth that occurs in children if they ingest too much fluoride during tooth development. Some studies report that in sensitive individuals fluoride damages the nervous and immune systems, possibly setting the stage for multiple chemical sensitivities. Fluoride also may interfere with various enzyme systems, harm a developing fetus, and play a role in arthritis, gastric ulcers, atherosclerosis, kidney disorders, and migraine headaches.

It is relatively easy to get too much fluoride, as it is found in soils, plants, animal tissues, water supplies, dental products, and fluoride vitamin supplements, as well as foods and beverages processed with fluoridated water. Moderate fluorosis occurs in 1% to 2% of children exposed to 1 ppm (parts per million) fluoride and in approximately 10% of children exposed to 2 ppm. Moderate to severe fluorosis occurs in varying percentages up to as high as 33% of children exposed to 2.4 to 4.1 ppm.

The groups at potentially higher risk for fluoride-associated problems consist of formula-fed infants, heavy exercisers (because they consume more fluoridated water), individuals with high consumption of water-based beverages, people with malfunctioning kidneys, and elderly people.

■ RDA AND DOSAGE

No RDA has been established for fluoride. The U.S. Environmental Protection Agency's suggested range for fluoride in municipal water supplies is 0.7 to 1.2 ppm. The maximal acceptable limit is 4 ppm.

■ FOOD SOURCES

Fluoride content varies widely in soils, water, plants, and animals in different areas of the United States. Many cities have fluoridated water supplies, but more and more people are coming to believe that municipal water supplies contain unacceptably high levels of toxins and opt for bottled or filtered water, which does not contain fluoride. Fluoride also is available in toothpastes, mouthwashes, topical dental applications, fluoride vitamin supplements, and foods processed with fluoridated water.

FOLIC ACID (FOLACIN)

Drugs that deplete folic acid (folacin)

■ AMILORIDE	■ ESTROGENS,	DICLOFENAC,
■ ALUMINUM-	CONJUGATED	FENOPROFEN,
CONTAINING ANTACIDS	■ ESTROGENS,	IBUPROFEN,
■ ASPIRIN	ESTERIFIED	KETOPROFEN,
■ BARBITURATES	■ ETHSUXIMIDE	NAPROXEN)
■ CARBAMAZEPINE	■ FAMOTIDINE	■ ORAL CONTRACEPTIVES
■ CHOLESTYRAMINE	■ FOSPHENYTOIN	■ PHENOBARTIBAL
■ CHOLINE MAGNESIUM	■ HYDROCHLORTHIAZIDE	■ PHENYTOIN
TRISALICYLATE	AND TRIAMTERENE	■ PRIMIDONE
■ CHOLINE SALICYLATE	■ INDOMETHACIN	■ RANITIDINE
■ CIMETIDINE	■ MAGNESIUM-	■ SALSALATE
■ CO-TRIMOXAZOLE	CONTAINING ANTACIDS	■ SULFASALAZINE
■ COLESTIPOL	■ METFORMIN	■ TRIAMTERENE
■ CORTICOSTEROIDS	■ METHOTREXATE	■ TRIMETHOPRIM
■ COX-2 INHIBITORS	■ NIZATIDINE	■ VALPROIC ACID AND
(INCLUDES CELECOXIB	■ NONSTEROIDAL ANTI-	DERIVATIVES
AND ROFECOXIB)	INFLAMMATORY DRUGS	■ ZONISAMIDE
■ CYCLOSERINE	(INCLUDING	
■ DIFLUNISAL	ETODOLAC,	

FOLIC ACID is a member of the B vitamin group. Isolated in 1946 from spinach leaves, its name comes from *folium*, the Latin word for leaf. In the body, folic acid is converted to its biologically active form, tetrahydrofolic acid (THFA). Niacin and vitamin C are necessary for this conversion. Structurally, folic acid consists of a pteridine (containing two rings) nucleus, conjugated with para-aminobenzoic acid, and glutamic acid. Hence, its chemical name is pteroylmonoglutamate.

■ SYMPTOMS AND CAUSES OF DEFICIENCY

A deficiency in folic acid disrupts DNA metabolism, which causes abnormal cellular development, especially in red blood cells, white blood cells, and cells of the stomach, intestine, vagina, and cervix. The need for folic acid is greater during pregnancy.

Folic acid is one of the most commonly deficient vitamins. Heat, light, and oxygen easily destroy it, so destruction of folic acid occurs during food processing, cooking, and storage.[7] One study reported that cooking can destroy virtually all the free folic acid in foods.

Folic acid deficiency can result in megaloblastic anemia, birth defects, cervical dysplasia, elevated homocysteine, headache, fatigue, depression, hair loss, anorexia, insomnia, diarrhea, nausea, infections, and increased rates of breast and colorectal cancers. More recently, folic acid deficiency has been reported to increase the risk for breast cancer and colorectal cancer. Many drugs have been shown to deplete folic acid. Three of the major conditions are elaborated upon below.

• *Anemia:* Folic acid is required for the production of red blood cells, which carry oxygen from the lungs to the tissues and carbon dioxide from the tissues to the lungs. A deficiency in folic acid causes anemia and reduced oxygenation of tissues. This results in a condition known as megaloblastic anemia, characterized by enlarged, abnormal red blood cells. This condition can produce tiredness, weakness, diarrhea, and weight loss.

• *Birth defects:* Folic acid helps regulate the development of nerves and the transfer of genetic material to new cells. During pregnancy, the rapidly growing fetus increases a woman's need for folic acid substantially, and a folic acid deficiency during pregnancy dramatically increases the risk for birth defects such as spina bifida and cleft palate. The link between folic acid deficiency and birth defects is so strong that all women of childbearing age are advised to have their folic acid status checked before trying to become pregnant. Following this practice probably would prevent thousands of birth defects each year. A laboratory test, the Neutrophilic Hypersegmentation Index (NHI), can easily identify the earliest stages of folate insufficiency.

• *Cervical dysplasia:* The development of abnormal cells in the uterus, cervical dysplasia is regarded as a precancerous condition that usually is discovered when a woman has a Pap exam. This condition may contribute to an increased number of hysterectomies. More than 800,000 women have hysterectomies every year in the United States. Some health care professionals believe that the folic acid depletion caused by oral contraceptives and other medications is linked to this high incidence of cervical dysplasia and hysterectomies.

• *Elevated homocysteine,* also known as hyperhomocysteinemia, is now recognized as a serious risk factor for cardiovascular disease. Excessive homocysteine is capable of directly damaging the cells in the lining of arteries, which causes plaque build-up and atherosclerosis. Even moderate elevations of homocysteine represent a substantially increased risk for the development of plaque build-up and blood clots.

■ BIOLOGICAL FUNCTIONS AND EFFECTS

The following list outlines the many biological functions of folic acid:

• Like vitamin B_{12}, folic acid is intimately involved in the synthesis of both DNA and RNA. Hence, it is essential for proper cell division and the transmission of one's genetic code to all newly formed cells.

• Folic acid may protect against certain types of cancers including: (a) precancerous cervical dysplasia in women (especially those taking oral contraceptives), (b) bronchial squamous metaplasia in long-time heavy cigarette smokers, (c) dysplasia associated with ulcerative colitis and colon cancer, and (d) breast cancer.

• Folic acid prevents birth abnormalities such as neural tube defects, cleft palate, and cleft lip.

• Folic acid is essential for the healthy maturation of red cells and white blood cells.

• Folic acid supplementation has been shown to prevent cervical dysplasia, a precancerous condition.

• Folic acid is required for the conversion of homocysteine to methionine. High blood levels of homocysteine are associated with the development of atherosclerosis.

• Folic acid is synthesized by the "friendly" intestinal bacteria.

■ SYMPTOMS OF TOXICITY

Although folic acid is essentially nontoxic, even at high doses, large doses of folic acid can mask an underlying vitamin B_{12} deficiency. If undetected, this deficiency could result in irreversible nerve damage. Consequently, folic acid is limited to 800 mcg in over-the-counter nutritional supplements.

■ RDA AND DOSAGE

The RDA for folic acid is 200 mcg/day. Pregnant and lactating women require dosages higher than the RDA. Pharmacologic dosages in the scientific literature range from 400 mcg up to 5000 mcg.

■ FOOD SOURCES

Folic acid is found in a wide variety of foods. Best sources are dark green leafy vegetables, brewer's yeast, liver, and eggs. Other good sources are beets, broccoli, Brussels sprouts, orange juice, cabbage, cauliflower, cantaloupe, kidney and lima beans, wheat germ, and whole-grain cereals and breads.

INOSITOL

Drugs that deplete inositol		
■ AMINOGLYCOSIDES	■ MACROLIDES	■ TETRACYCLINES
■ CEPHALOSPORINS	■ PENICILLINS	■ TRIMETHOPRIM
■ FLUOROQUINOLONES	■ SULFONAMIDES	■ ZONISAMIDE

ALTHOUGH INOSITOL has been recognized for a long time, scientists first realized it was a vitamin in 1940. Inositol is a sugar-like, water-soluble substance that is a member of the B vitamin complex. It is found in the liver, kidney, skeleton, and heart muscle. In animal tissues, inositol is a component of phospholipids, and in plants it usually occurs as phytic acid. In humans, inositol is synthesized in the intestinal tract by the "friendly" bacteria.

■ SYMPTOMS AND CAUSES OF DEFICIENCY

No inositol deficiency has been identified in humans, and a deficiency is not likely because of its widespread occurrence in foods.

■ BIOLOGICAL FUNCTIONS AND EFFECTS

Inositol is an essential component of phospholipids in cellular membranes of animals and humans. The metabolically active form of inositol is myoinositol, which occurs abundantly in muscle tissue. As part of phospholipids in cellular membranes, phosphatidylinositol helps to mediate cellular responses to external stimuli. Phosphatidylinositol also facilitates the production of arachidonic acid.

Several studies have shown that inositol can be effective in treating depression, panic, and obsessive–compulsive disorders. Myoinositol may be helpful in the treatment of diabetic neuropathy.

■ SIDE EFFECTS AND TOXICITY

No toxicity has been reported or observed for inositol.

■ RDA AND DOSAGE

No RDA has been set for inositol. Pharmacologic doses in the scientific literature range from 100 mg to 1000 mg.

■ FOOD SOURCES

Myoinositol occurs in foods in three different forms: free myoinositol, phytic acid, and inositol-containing phospholipids. The richest sources of myoinositol are the seeds of plants such as beans, grains, and nuts. The richest animal sources are organ meats. Free myoinositol predominates in the brain and kidneys, whereas phospholipid-inositol is concentrated in skeletal muscle, heart, liver, and pancreas. Humans also consume phytic acid, or inositol hexaphosphate, a common component of plant cells.

IODINE

Drugs that deplete iodine

NO KNOWN STUDIES HAVE REPORTED DRUG-INDUCED IODINE DEPLETIONS.

THE ONLY KNOWN FUNCTION of iodine is the role it plays in the thyroid hormones diiodotyrosine, triiodothryonine (T_3), and thyroxin (T_4). Dietary iodine is converted to iodide in the intestinal tract, where it is easily absorbed and transported to the thyroid gland. In the thyroid gland, iodine is stored in a protein complex called thyroglobulin.

Iodine metabolism and thyroid hormone production are regulated by a hormonal control system. A decline in blood thyroid hormones triggers the hypothalamus to release thyroid-releasing hormone (TRH), which in turn signals the pituitary gland to release thyroid-stimulating hormone (TSH). An increase in TSH stimulates the thyroid gland to increase the uptake of iodine and synthesize more thyroid hormones. TSH also stimulates the thyroid gland to produce enzymes that release the thyroid hormones into circulation for delivery to cells throughout the body.

■ SYMPTOMS AND CAUSES OF DEFICIENCY

A deficiency of iodine can produce the following conditions:

• *Hypothyroidism:* A lack of iodine decreases thyroid hormone synthesis. The lower thyroid activity reduces the rate of energy production. Manifestations of hypothyroidism include fatigue and weight gain.

• *Goiter:* A deficiency of iodine can result in enlargement of the thyroid gland. When this becomes visible, it is called a simple goiter. Symptoms of goiter include dry skin and hair, brittle nails, constipation, fatigue, depression, weight gain, and difficulty in swallowing.

The condition can be prevented, and it is frequently cured by administering iodine.

• *Cretinism:* Iodine deficiency during pregnancy can cause cretinism in the developing fetus, a severe condition characterized by both mental and physical retardation.

• *Myxedema:* Iodine deficiency is one of the causes of myxedema. The resulting hypofunction (lower function) of the thyroid gland causes a slower metabolic rate, anemia, enlarged tongue, slow speech, puffiness of the hands and face, problems with the skin and hair, drowsiness, and mental apathy.

Goitrogens are naturally occurring substances in some foods that can inhibit the synthesis and secretion of thyroid hormones. Some common foods containing goitrogens are raw cabbage, turnips, cauliflower, soy beans, and peanuts. Problems are unlikely unless a person who is iodine-deficient consumes large amounts of these foods over a period of time. Cooking deactivates the goitrogen compounds in these foods.

■ BIOLOGICAL FUNCTIONS AND EFFECTS

The effects of iodine are all related to the activity and function of the hormones of the thyroid gland. The iodine-dependent thyroid hormones regulate cellular oxygen consumption, basal metabolism, and energy production throughout the body. As a result, the thyroid hormones control a variety of biological and physiological activities, including body temperature, physical growth, reproduction, neuromuscular function, the synthesis of proteins, and the growth of skin and hair.

Iodine deficiency may be a contributing factor to fibrocystic breasts. Iodine supplementation has caused complete relief of symptoms in some women.

Iodine-containing products such as SSKI (saturated solution of potassium iodide) and organidin are frequently effective for loosening up irritating mucous secretions. These mucolytic agents require a doctor's prescription.

If the thyroid gland is damaged or absent, the basal metabolic rate can decline to as low as 55% of normal, resulting in impaired growth and development.

When the thyroid gland is hyperactive, the basal metabolic rate can go up as high as 160% of normal, causing tachycardia, nervousness, and excitability.

■ SIDE EFFECTS AND TOXICITY

Iodine is a relatively benign trace element that generally causes no harm at dosages 10 to 20 times above normal daily needs. The thyroid gland absorbs more iodine, but thyroid synthesis remains normal.

Chronic excessive intake of iodine can cause enlargement of the thyroid gland resembling goiter. This condition is called "iodine goiter."

■ RDA AND DOSAGE

The RDA for iodine is 150 mcg/day. Pharmacologic doses for iodine in scientific studies are generally in the range of 3 mg to 6 mg/day.

■ FOOD SOURCES

The most common source of iodine in the United States is iodized salt. Iodine-rich foods include seafood, sea vegetables (seaweed), and vegetables grown in iodine-rich soils.

IRON

Drugs that deplete iron

■ ASPIRIN	■ CHOESTIPOL	■ PENICILLAMINE
■ CHOLESTYRAMINE	■ FAMOTIDINE	■ RANITIDINE
■ CHOLINE MAGNESIUM TRISALICYLATE	■ INDOMETHACIN	■ SALICYLATES
	■ LEVOTHYROXINE	■ STANOZOLOL
■ CHOLINE SALICYLATE	■ NEOMYCIN	■ TETRACYCLINES
■ CIMETIDINE	■ NIZATIDINE	

IRON plays a vital role in many biochemical pathways. It is involved in oxygen transport within blood and muscles, electron transfer in the cellular uptake of oxygen, and conversion of blood sugar to energy. Iron also is part of many enzymes involved with making new cells, amino acids, hormones, and neurotransmitters. In the body, iron exists in various functional forms (in hemoglobin and in enzymes) and in transport and storage forms (ferritin, transferrin, and hemosiderin).

■ SYMPTOMS AND CAUSES OF DEFICIENCY

About 80% of the iron in the body is in the blood, so iron loss is greatest whenever blood is lost. The most common cause of iron deficiency is the loss of iron through menstrual bleeding is. To replace their monthly losses, menstruating women require approximately twice as much iron intake as men.

Individuals at risk for iron deficiency include infants, adolescent girls, pregnant women, menstruating women, and people with bleeding ulcers. Vegetarians are at risk for anemia because the main dietary source of iron is from meat/animal protein foods.

Iron-deficiency anemia is the classic condition in which red blood cells contain less than optimum hemoglobin and consequently carry less oxygen.

Symptoms of iron-deficiency anemia are weakness, fatigue, skin pallor, headache, hair loss, labored breathing after exertion, spooning (inversion) of fingernails, brittle nails, and greater susceptibility to infections. Additional related conditions include the following.

- Deliberately consuming large quantities of ice, called pagophagia, is related to iron deficiency and is completely resolved with low-level iron supplementation.

- Hypochlorhydria, low production of hydrochloric acid in the stomach, causes decreased iron absorption. Low production of hydrochloric acid occurs often in the elderly and can lead to iron-deficiency anemia.

- Antacids and drugs that alter gastric acidity inhibit iron absorption.

- Complexing agents, such as phytates, oxalates, and phosphates, form insoluble iron complexes, which reduce absorption.

- Vitamin E inhibits the absorption of iron. Although taking vitamin E generally is not a cause of iron deficiency, it is not advisable to take supplemental doses of iron and vitamin E at the same time.

- Diarrhea, intestinal inflammation, and other conditions that increase intestinal motility reduce absorption.

- Iron deficiency can cause hair loss.

- Athletes tend to be more susceptible to iron loss because their level of activity utilizes more iron stores.

■ BIOLOGICAL FUNCTIONS AND EFFECTS

The functions of iron in the body are summarized as follows.

- The major function of iron is for oxygen transport by hemoglobin, the oxygen-carrying protein in red blood cells. The heme portion of hemoglobin contains four atoms of iron. Iron picks up the oxygen in the lungs, where the concentration is high. Iron binds the oxygen and then transports it to the tissues and releases it wherever it is needed.

- Myoglobin is an iron-containing protein in muscles that accepts oxygen and serves as an oxygen storage reservoir in muscle.

- Iron is one of the substances necessary for optimal immune response.

- Iron is necessary for the synthesis of the amino acid carnitine, which plays an essential role in the metabolism of fatty acids.

- Much of the functional activity of iron in electron transport and energy production has to do with its ability to convert back and forth between its reduced or ferrous state (Fe^{++}) and its oxidized ferric state (Fe^{+++}).

- Iron plays an important role in liver detoxification enzymes, which remove toxins from the body.
- Iron is part of the enzymes that initiate the synthesis of the neurotransmitters serotonin and dopamine.
- The synthesis of collagen and elastin require iron.

■ SIDE EFFECTS AND TOXICITY

When the body's iron stores are full, the body absorbs less iron. Therefore, iron toxicity is rare, but it can occur. The primary causes of iron toxicity are:

- Ingesting too much iron.
- A genetic defect called hemochromatosis, usually occurring in men, which causes excessive iron absorption, resulting in damage to the heart, liver, spleen and pancreas.
- Alcoholism, which can cause intestinal and liver damage leading to increased iron absorption.

■ RDA AND DOSAGE

The RDA for iron is 15 mg/day for women and 10 mg/day for men. Pharmacologic doses in the scientific literature range from 10 mg/day to 50 mg/day.

Available forms are ferrous sulfate, ferrous gluconate, ferrous fumerate, ferrous glycinate, and ferric ammonium citrate.

■ FOOD SOURCES

Liver is by far the richest iron-containing food. Additional good animal sources of iron-rich foods are other organ meats, fish, and poultry.

The best plant sources of iron are dried beans and vegetables, followed by dried fruits, nuts, and whole-grain breads and cereals. Fortified cereals, flours, and breads with iron have contributed significantly to daily consumption of dietary iron.

LACTOBACILLUS ACIDOPHILUS

Drugs that deplete Lactobacillus acidophilus

■ AMINOGLYCOSIDES	■ FLUOROQUINOLONES	■ SULFONAMIDES
■ CEPHALOSPORINS	■ MACROLIDES	■ TETRACYCLINES
■ CO-TRIMOXAZOLE	■ PENICILLINS	

LACTOBACILLUS ACIDOPHILUS is the primary strain of beneficial or "friendly" bacteria that inhabit the small intestine. If the balance between the beneficial and the pathological bacteria is upset, a condition known as dysbiosis develops. The use of antibiotics is the most common cause of dysbiosis because antibiotics kill most of the acidophilus bacteria along with the pathological bacteria.

Maintaining a healthy colonization of intestinal microflora with beneficial bacteria such as *L. acidophilus* is a key factor in maintaining a healthy immune system. Products containing beneficial bacteria are frequently referred to as probiotics.

■ SYMPTOMS AND CAUSES OF DEFICIENCY

A deficiency of *L. acidophilus* bacteria can result in the growth and proliferation of pathological organisms in the intestinal tract. This can decrease digestion and absorption of nutrients, as well as increase production of gas, bloating, and toxins.

The most common cause of a deficiency of *L. acidophilus* bacteria is the use of antibiotic drugs. Other factors that can cause a reduction of *L. acidophilus* include the use of drugs that increase intestinal pH, stress, diarrhea, intestinal infections, high-sugar/low-fiber diets, and toxins in the intestine.

A deficiency of *L. acidophilus* bacteria can result in the proliferation of pathological organisms in the intestinal tract. This can decrease digestion and absorption of nutrients, as well as increase production of gas, bloating, and toxins.

■ BIOLOGICAL FUNCTIONS AND EFFECTS

The following are functions and effects of *L. acidophilus*:

• *Lactobacillus acidophilus* bacteria act as a barrier against infection by producing natural antibiotics in the intestinal tract that to inhibit the growth of more than twenty types of harmful bacteria.

• The metabolism of *L. acidophilus* bacteria produces lactic acid and hydrogen peroxide, which together create an environment unfavorable for the growth of yeasts and other harmful bacteria.

• *L. acidophilus* bacteria promote healthy digestion by producing enzymes that help to digest fats, proteins, and dairy products.

• *L. acidophilus* organisms produce a wide range of B vitamins and vitamin K in the intestinal tract.

• Oral ingestion of acidophilus has been shown to enhance the activity of the immune system throughout the whole body.

• *L. acidophilus* bacteria metabolize cholesterol, so they can help to lower elevated cholesterol levels and thereby reduce the risk of cardiovascular disease.

■ SIDE EFFECTS AND TOXICITY

L. acidophilus has no known toxic effects, and these beneficial bacteria do not interfere with other medications.

■ RDA AND DOSAGE

No RDA has been set for *Lactobacillus acidophilus*. Dosages for probiotics are measured in of cfu's (colony forming units), which denotes the number of live organisms per dose.

The dosage range for prevention in healthy people is from 1 to 2 billion cfu per day. For patients who have dysbiosis and those who have been taking antibiotics, the recommended range is 10–15 billion cfu twice daily (with food) for 2 weeks.

■ FOOD SOURCES

Small amounts of *L. acidophilus* occur in cultured food products such as yogurt and acidophilus milk. To be effective therapeutically, however, larger quantities should be consumed in the form of probiotic supplements.

MAGNESIUM

Drugs that deplete magnesium

■ AMINOGLYCOSIDES	■ DIGOXIN	■ INDAPAMIDE
■ AMPHOTERICIN B	■ ESTROGENS,	■ METOLAZONE
■ BENZTHIAZIDE	CONJUGATED	■ ORAL CONTRACEPTIVES
■ BUMETANIDE	■ ESTROGENS,	■ PENICILLAMINE
■ CHLOROTHIAZIDE	ESTERIFIED	■ PENTAMIDINE
■ CHLOROTRIANISENE	■ ETHACRYNIC ACID	■ POLYTHIAZIDE
■ CHOLESTYRAMINE	■ FOSCARNET	■ QUINESTROL
■ CHLORTHALIDONE	■ FUROSEMIDE	■ QUINETHAZONE
■ CORTICOSTEROIDS	■ HYDROCHLORO-	■ TETRACYCLINES
■ CYCLOSERINE	THIAZIDE	■ TORSEMIDE
■ DIETHYLSTILBESTEROL	■ HYDROFLUMETHIAZIDE	■ TRICHLORMETHIAZIDE

MAGNESIUM is a co-factor in more than 300 enzymatic reactions in the body. This mineral is necessary for the transmission of nerve impulses, muscular activity, temperature regulation, detoxification reactions, and the formation of healthy bones and teeth. It also plays a crucial role in energy production and in the synthesis of DNA and RNA.

A survey taken by the U.S. Department of Agriculture revealed that approximately 75% of Americans do not ingest the RDA of magnesium, making it one of the most commonly deficient nutrients in the United States.[8] Less than optimal magnesium intake compromises all tissues, especially tissues of the heart, nerves, and kidneys.

Magnesium is an extremely important nutrient for the cardiovascular system. A deficiency is associated with an increased incidence of atherosclerosis, hypertension, strokes, and heart attacks. Low levels of magnesium can cause stiffness in the blood vessels, which elevates blood pressure, and a contraction or spasm in the heart muscle, which can result in sudden death. Many heart attacks occur in individuals with a relatively healthy heart, and a magnesium deficiency is the instigator of the heart spasm that results in death.

Magnesium singlehandedly influences many of the activities associated with a wide variety of cardiac medications. For example, magnesium inhibits platelet aggregation (like aspirin), thins the blood (like Coumadin), blocks calcium uptake (like calcium channel-blocking drugs such as Procardia), and relaxes blood vessels (like ACE inhibitors such as Vasotec). Magnesium also increases oxygenation of the heart muscle by improving the heart's ability to contract.

■ SYMPTOMS AND CAUSES OF DEFICIENCY

Although a critical deficiency of magnesium is rare in the United States, a marginal deficiency seems to be widespread. Some studies report that approximately 75% of Americans ingest less than the RDA. Deficiency symptoms include muscle cramps, weakness, insomnia, loss of appetite, intestinal disorders, kidney stones, osteoporosis, nervousness, restlessness, irritability, fear, anxiety, confusion, depression, fatigue, and high blood pressure. Magnesium depletion creates an elevated calcium-to-magnesium ratio, which can precipitate a cardiac muscle spasm resulting in a heart attack and, frequently, death.

Causes of magnesium depletion in the body are as follows:

• Food processing is a major cause of magnesium depletion. For example, up to 85% of magnesium is lost when whole wheat is refined to produce white flour.

• Artificial fertilizers used in modern farming techniques contribute to the depletion of magnesium in the soil and usually do not contain any magnesium to replace it.

• Poor food choices, including excess calcium can cause a deficiency of magnesium.

• Intestinal malabsorption is sometimes a factor in deficient magnesium.

• Alcohol abuse, liver and kidney diseases can be causal factors.

• Diabetes can cause deficiencies. Hypomagnesemia occurs in approximately 25% of patients with diabetes. Low levels of magnesium have been reported in childhood Type I diabetes and in adults with Type I or Type II diabetes.

■ BIOLOGICAL FUNCTIONS AND EFFECTS

In general, magnesium is required for the metabolism of carbohydrates, proteins, and fats, as well as activity related to calcium, phosphorus, and vitamin C. Magnesium is vital to the health of nervous and muscular tissues throughout the body. Specific functions and effects of magnesium in the body are summarized as follows:

- Magnesium influences many aspects of cardiovascular health. It acts to decrease platelet aggregation.
- stickiness, helps to thin the blood, blocks calcium uptake, and relaxes blood vessels.
- Adequate magnesium intake reduces the risk of cardiovascular disease and increases the rate of survival following a heart attack. Administering intravenous magnesium in early stages of a heart attack results in a 70% decrease in deaths within one month following the event.
- More than thirty clinical trials have reported that magnesium can lower high blood pressure. The effect usually is only moderate, however. Therefore, magnesium should not be viewed as a primary treatment for hypertension.
- Many studies report that women with premenstrual syndrome (PMS) have low levels of magnesium. Some studies report that magnesium helps to relieve PMS symptoms.
- Various studies report low magnesium levels in asthma patients. Consuming adequate magnesium may reduce the risk of developing asthma and frequently is used as part of an overall treatment program.
- Magnesium is extremely important for bone health. It is involved in calcium metabolism, the synthesis of vitamin D, and the integrity of skeletal bone-crystal formation.
- Magnesium helps to bind calcium to tooth enamel, thereby creating an effective barrier to tooth decay.

■ SIDE EFFECTS AND TOXICITY

Because the kidneys excrete excess magnesium, magnesium toxicity is rare. Excess magnesium intake frequently causes diarrhea.

■ RDA AND DOSAGE

The RDA for magnesium is 400 mg/day. Pharmacologic doses in the scientific literature range from 500 mg to 1,500 mg/day.

Available forms include magnesium oxide, hydroxide, gluconate, glycinate, sulfate, chloride, aspartate, malate, succinate, fumarate, ascorbate, and citrate.

■ FOOD SOURCES

Magnesium content in foods varies widely, as does its content in soil. Good food sources include:

- nuts
- legumes
- cereal grains
- dark green leafy vegetables

MANGANESE

Drugs that deplete manganese

NO STUDIES REPORTING DRUG-INDUCED MANGANESE DEPLETION HAVE BEEN FOUND.

MANGANESE is a co-factor that aids in the activation of a wide variety of enzymes. Manganese-containing enzymes influence many biological activities, including the synthesis of collagen, protein, mucopolysaccharides, cholesterol, and fatty acids. It also is necessary for the normal growth of bones and the metabolism of amino acids.

The average human body contains only about 20 mg of manganese, most of which is stored in the bones. Smaller amounts are concentrated in the pituitary gland, liver, pancreas, and intestinal mucus. Absorption takes place throughout the entire small intestine.

■ SYMPTOMS AND CAUSES OF DEFICIENCY

Manganese deficiency in humans is relatively uncommon because the mineral magnesium is capable of substituting for manganese in many of the enzyme-related functions of manganese. The following are specific manifestations of deficiency:

- The most notable symptoms of manganese deficiency are skeletal abnormalities such as loss of muscle coordination, propensity for sprains and strains, and weak ligaments. These problems develop as a result of the reduced synthesis of collagen and mucopolysaccharides.

- Manganese deficiency impairs glucose metabolism and produces abnormalities in the secretion of insulin.

- Low manganese levels often are found in people with epilepsy, hypoglycemia, schizophrenia, and osteoporosis. Women with osteoporosis have been shown to have low levels of manganese.

- Manganese is necessary for the biosynthesis of cholesterol, and hypocholesterolemia may be associated with manganese deficiency.

- Intestinal absorption is hindered by ingesting manganese in large amounts, in which case the effect is great. In small amounts, the effect is small or negligible.

■ BIOLOGICAL FUNCTIONS AND EFFECTS

The major functions of manganese in the body are summarized as follows:

• Manganese is necessary for the production of mucopolysaccharides, glycoproteins, and lipopolysaccharides, which are necessary for the growth and maintenance of connective tissue and cartilage.

• In conjunction with vitamin K, manganese plays a role in the synthesis of prothrombin and the regulation of blood-clotting.

• Manganese influences the activity of osteoblasts and osteoclasts, which makes this mineral essential for normal bone growth and development.

• Manganese is the central metal co-factor in mitochondrial superoxide dismutase, and as such, it is essential for optimal functioning of one of the body's most important antioxidant defense systems, protecting against the toxic effects of oxygen during energy production.

• Manganese is necessary in the synthesis of thyroxine, the principal hormone of the thyroid gland.

• Manganese is involved with the production of dopamine and melanin and in the synthesis of fatty acids.

■ SIDE EFFECTS AND TOXICITY

Manganese is safe, and people can tolerate relatively large oral doses with no apparent adverse effects. Miners have developed toxicity to manganese after inhaling manganese dust in the course of their work.

Toxicity can produce dementia, psychiatric disorders resembling schizophrenia, and neurologic disorders resembling Parkinson's disease.

■ RDA AND DOSAGE

The safe and adequate range for manganese is from 2 to 5 mg/day. Pharmacologic doses range from 2 to 50 mg/day.

■ FOOD SOURCES

Manganese is widely distributed in foods of plant and animal origin. The best food sources include:

• whole-grain breads and cereals   • vegetables
• nuts   • raisins
• dried beans and peas   • pineapple

MELATONIN

MELATONIN is a naturally occurring hormone that regulates sleep. It is secreted by the pineal gland in the brain. The body's level of melatonin declines with aging. Adults experience about a 37% decline in daily melatonin output between 20 and 70 years of age, with most of the decline occurring after age 40.[9]

The output of melatonin is regulated by the amount of light that enters our eyes. Melatonin products are available as sublingual (fast-acting) tablets, regular tablets or capsules, and timed-release (long-acting) products. The sublingual form is best for people who have trouble falling asleep. The timed-release products work better with individuals who wake up during the night.

■ SYMPTOMS AND CAUSES OF DEFICIENCY

Insomnia and other sleep disturbances are the primary symptoms of melatonin deficiency. A deficiency of vitamin B_6 can inhibit the synthesis of serotonin, and subsequently the conversion of serotonin to melatonin. Therefore, all drugs that deplete vitamin B_6 (see page 56–57) can potentially inhibit the synthesis of melatonin and cause insomnia.

Research in human cell cultures and with animals indicates that melatonin may provide protection against certain types of cancer. Low levels of melatonin could constitute an increased risk for breast cancer. One possible explanation has to do with melatonin's antioxidant activity. Thus, a melatonin deficiency could result in increased levels of free radical damage, which could lead to cancer.

■ BIOLOGICAL FUNCTIONS AND EFFECTS

The functions and effects of melatonin related to sleep can be summarized as follows:

• Melatonin is a master control hormone that regulates our 24-hour circadian rhythm.

• The primary function of melatonin seems to be its role in regulating the sleep/wake cycle. When darkness falls, melatonin levels rise, which triggers the sleep cycle.

• Melatonin has been used successfully to treat jet lag.

Also, melatonin possesses important antioxidant activity. And melatonin controls the output of growth hormone and the sex hormones.

■ RDA AND DOSAGE

No RDA has been set for melatonin. Common nighttime dosages range from 0.5 mg to 3.0 mg. Dosages for specific therapeutic applications can be much higher.

Melatonin is available in sublingual (fast-acting) tablets, regular tablets or capsules, and timed-release forms.

■ SIDE EFFECTS AND TOXICITY

Melatonin seems to be safe and nontoxic. To date, however, long-term studies have not been conducted with humans. Taking too much melatonin can cause morning grogginess and undesired drowsiness at other times of day.

■ FOOD SOURCES

Melatonin does not occur in foods in any significant amount.

MOLYBDENUM

Drugs that deplete molybdenum

NO STUDIES THAT REPORT DRUG-INDUCED MOLYBDENUM DEFICIENCY HAVE BEEN LOCATED.

EVEN THOUGH MOLYBDENUM is one of the rarest substances on earth, small amounts of this mineral are found in all tissues of the human body. Molybdenum is a component of several important metalloenzymes that participate in liver detoxification. Most biochemistry textbooks acknowledge that little is known about this trace mineral beyond its role as a co-factor for several enzymes.

■ SYMPTOMS AND CAUSES OF DEFICIENCY

Molybdenum deficiency in humans is rare because so little is needed. In a healthy state, body tissues contain less than 0.1 parts per million.

Molybdenum co-factor deficiency syndrome is a rare genetic condition characterized by seizures and developmental delays in newborns. A deficiency of molybdenum is found occasionally in individuals who have been receiving prolonged total parenteral nutrition (TPN). Symptoms include tachycardia, headache, mental disturbances, and coma.

Increased intake of sulfate or copper can cause excessive excretion of molybdenum.

■ Biological Functions and Effects

The complex functions of molybdenum are summarized as follows:

- Molybdenum is necessary for the function of three enzymes: xanthine oxidase, aldehyde oxidase, and sulfite oxidase.
- Xanthine oxidase metabolizes xanthine to uric acid for urinary excretion.
- Uric acid usually is considered to be a negative substance because of its association with gouty arthritis. At certain levels, however, uric acid is a powerful antioxidant that neutralizes free radicals. Thus, molybdenum may help regulate important antioxidant functions.
- Sulfite oxidase catalyzes the last step in the metabolism of sulfur-containing amino acids. It enables the conversion to sulfite (which is toxic to the nervous system) to sulfate for excretion.
- Molybdenum affects the absorption of iron, copper, and sulfate.
- Aldehyde oxidase catalyzes the conversion of aldehydes to acids.

■ Side Effects and Toxicity

Molybdenum toxicity is rare. An excessive intake (10 to 15 mg/day) can cause a gout-like syndrome resulting from excess production of uric acid.

■ RDA and Dosage

The National Academy of Sciences has determined that a reasonable dietary level of molybdenum is between 10 and 500 mcg/day. Pharmacologic doses in the scientific literature range from 100 to 1000 mcg/day.

■ Food Sources

Good food sources of molybdenum are whole grains, organ meats, leafy green vegetables, legumes, and beans.

The availability of molybdenum varies widely according to the molybdenum content of the soil. Vegetables grown in molybdenum-rich soil can contain up to 500 times more molybdenum than those grown in molybdenum-deficient soils.

NICKEL

Drugs that deplete nickel

No studies that report drug-induced depletion of nickel have been found.

IN 1974, NICKEL was discovered to be an essential nutrient in baby chicks. Since then, it has been found to have an essential physiological role in the metabolism of other animals including humans. Its functions, however, are still far from being understood at this time.

Nickel is present in the blood, various organs, teeth, bone, skin, and the brain of humans, with the largest concentrations found in the skin and the bone marrow. Nickel is so ubiquitous in nature (it occurs in air, plants, and animals) that scientists have only recently been able to effectively prepare nickel-deficient diets so the biological effects of this mineral could begin to be tested. To date, more is known about the effects of nickel in various animals than in humans.

■ SYMPTOMS AND CAUSES OF DEFICIENCY

Nickel is so common in the environment that deficiency is rare.
From studies in animals:

- Low levels of nickel are associated with smaller litter sizes.

- Nickel deficiency causes abnormal changes in the livers of laboratory animals.

- Rats raised on nickel-deficient diets develop anemia related to a reduction in iron absorption.

■ BIOLOGICAL FUNCTIONS AND EFFECTS

The biological activities of nickel are thought to involve hormone, lipid (fat), and cellular membrane metabolism. Some specific functions are the following:

- Nickel has been found to be present normally in ribonucleic acid (RNA).

- Studies with rabbits and dogs have shown that nickel increases the hypoglycemic effect of insulin.

- Nickel is part of a protein called nickeloplasmin that is synthesized in the liver.

- Serum concentrations of nickel increase in response to stressful situations, such as a heart attack, a stroke, and even in women during the labor of childbirth.

- Nickel concentrations have been shown to influence the levels of a number of mitochondrial and liver enzymes.

■ SIDE EFFECTS AND TOXICITY

Under normal conditions, nickel is not a toxic element. Under less typical circumstances, nickel can produce some side effects, as follows:

- Nickel sensitivity from jewelry is relatively common in people who get their ears pierced.

- Some individuals with the skin conditions of psoriasis and eczema have been found to have elevated levels of nickel in the blood and skin.
- Occasionally in industry, nickel combines with carbon monoxide to form a toxic compound called nickel carbonyl. Industrial exposure to this compound has caused hospitalizations and several deaths.
- Excess exposure to or ingestion of nickel and nickel carbonyl is suspected to cause cancer. These compounds are found in tobacco and cigarette smoke.
- Inhalation of large quantities of certain nickel compounds has been shown to cause lung cancer in laboratory animals.
- Long-term intake of excessive nickel causes degeneration of the heart, brain, lungs, liver, and kidney.

■ RDA AND DOSAGE

Nickel has no RDA. It is so ubiquitous in the environment that studies on its supplementation have not been conducted.

■ FOOD SOURCES

Grains and vegetables are the best dietary sources of nickel. Animal foods are relatively poor sources of nickel.

PHOSPHORUS

Drugs that deplete phosphorus

■ ALUMINUM HYDROXIDE-CONTAINING MEDICATIONS	■ CHOLESTYRAMINE ■ COLCHICINE ■ DIGOXIN	■ MAGNESIUM-CONTAINING COMPOUNDS

PHOSPHORUS is the second most abundant mineral in the human body (calcium is the first). Approximately 80% of phosphorus is present in the skeleton, and the other 20% is active metabolically and plays a role in the metabolism of every cell in the body. In fact, phosphorus participates in more biological processes than any other mineral. A complete discussion of its functions would require delving into virtually every metabolic process in the body.

■ SYMPTOMS AND CAUSES OF DEFICIENCY

Although phosphorus deficiency has been reported in animals, it is rare in humans. Long-term use of aluminum-containing antacids could lead to phosphate depletion.

Individuals who might be at risk for phosphorus depletion include alcoholics, people with kidney malfunction, individuals with intestinal malabsorption syndromes such as celiac disease and Crohn's disease, and individuals on near-starvation diets.

■ BIOLOGICAL FUNCTIONS AND EFFECTS

Phosphorus and calcium form the insoluble calcium phosphate crystals that provide the strength and rigidity in bones and teeth. Unlike calcium, though, phosphorus is an integral part of the structure of soft tissues. As part of phospholipids, such as phosphatidylcholine, phosphorus is a component of all cellular membranes. Phosphorus is part of DNA and RNA and thus is necessary for all cellular reproduction and protein synthesis.

In addition:

- ATP contains three phosphate groups that are an essential part of energy storage and production processes in every cell throughout the body.
- Phosphorus is a part of many coenzymes and is involved in a wide variety of enzymatic reactions.
- In the form of phosphoric acid and its salts, phosphorus is part of one of the body's major buffer systems, which keep the pH or acidic/alkaline balance in the blood.

■ SIDE EFFECTS AND TOXICITY

Excessive consumption of foods high in phosphorus, such as animal protein and cola soft drinks, may inhibit calcium absorption and contribute to skeletal problems such as osteoporosis.

Excess phosphorus can produce hyperthyroidism, increase bone resorption, increase soft tissue calcium deposition, and decrease bone mass.

■ RDA AND DOSAGE

The RDA for phosphorus is 1000 mg/day. Higher dosages are not recommended. Most Americans consume far too much phosphorus.

■ FOOD SOURCES

Animal protein foods are the best source of phosphorus for most people. Cola soft drinks also contain a large amount of phosphorus.

POTASSIUM

Drugs that deplete potassium

- ACETAZOLAMIDE
- ALBUTEROL
- AMINOGLYCOSIDES
- AMPHOTERICIN B
- ASPIRIN
- BENZTHIAZIDE
- BISACODYL
- BUMETANIDE
- CHLOROTHIAZIDE
- CHOLINE MAGNESIUM TRISALICYLATE
- CHOLINE SALICYLATE

- COLCHICINE
- CORTICOSTEROIDS
- ETHACRYNIC ACID
- FOSCARNET
- FUROSEMIDE
- HYDROCHLORO-THIAZIDE
- HYDROFLUMETHIAZIDE
- INDAPAMIDE
- LEVODOPA
- METHYCLOTHIAZIDE

- METOLAZONE
- NIFEDIPINE
- PENICILLIN ANTIBIOTICS
- POLYTHIAZIDE
- QUINETHAZONE
- RITODRINE
- SODIUM BICARBONATE
- TERBUTALINE
- TORSEMIDE
- TRICHLORMETHIAZIDE
- VERAPAMIL

POTASSIUM is one of the body's three major electrolytes (the other two being sodium and chloride). They exist as fully dissociated ions and are the main particles responsible for osmotic pressure in body fluids. Potassium is the primary electrolyte functioning inside cells throughout the body. Their ionic strength enables them to influence the solubility of proteins and other substances throughout the body.

Hormonal control of potassium and the other electrolytes is mediated through the hormones of the adrenal cortex and the pituitary gland. Potassium is absorbed readily through the intestinal tract, and the excess is excreted efficiently in the urine via the kidneys.

■ SYMPTOMS AND CAUSES OF DEFICIENCY

In addition to the drugs mentioned, potassium deficiency can be caused by diarrhea, kidney failure, diabetic acidosis, and prolonged malnutrition vomiting. Other factors that can contribute to potassium depletion include use of alcohol or caffeine, excessive use of salt or sugar, and chronic stress.

Symptoms associated with potassium deficiency include irregular heartbeat, poor reflexes, muscle weakness, fatigue, continuous thirst, edema, constipation, dizziness, mental confusion, and nervous disorders.

■ BIOLOGICAL FUNCTIONS AND EFFECTS

Potassium plays essential roles in many of the body's most important functions, including nerve conduction, muscle contraction, and the beating of the heart. Specific functions and effects are the following:

- Potassium is the primary positively charged ion in intracellular fluids throughout the body. Approximately 98% of total body potassium resides inside cells.

- Potassium, along with sodium and chloride, helps to maintain normal osmotic equilibrium by controlling the distribution and balance of water throughout the body.
- Potassium controls the conduction of nerve impulses, maintenance of normal cardiac rhythm, and contraction of muscles.
- Potassium, in conjunction with other ions, helps to maintain the acid/alkaline balance throughout the body.
- Potassium has been shown to be effective in preventing hypertension and in some studies has been shown to help lower existing high blood pressure.
- Low levels of potassium are associated with increased risk for stroke.

One study reported that one serving of potassium-rich fruits or vegetables daily provided up to a 40% reduction in the risk of stroke.[10]

■ SIDE EFFECTS AND TOXICITY

Hyperkalemia (potassium toxicity) usually results from kidney failure, in which case blood levels rise because the kidneys cannot adequately excrete potassium. Malfunctioning adrenal glands also can cause hyperkalemia.

Symptoms of hyperkalemia include mental confusion, numbness of the extremities, labored breathing, and deteriorating heart activity.

■ RDA AND DOSAGE

No RDA has been established for potassium because it is so readily available in the diet. The estimated safe and adequate intake of potassium for adults is from 1.8 to 5.6 grams/day.

■ FOOD SOURCES

Potassium is plentiful in the diet. Potassium-rich foods include fresh fruits and vegetables, peanuts, meat, and milk. An average banana supplies more than 600 mg of potassium; half a cantaloupe contains 885 mg; 3 to 4 ounces of raw spinach contains about 775 mg; 2 ounces of peanuts contain about 575 mg; and one large, raw carrot contains about 330 mg.

S-ADENOSYL METHIONINE (SAME)

Drugs that deplete SAMe

■ LEVODOPA

SAME IS A METABOLITE of the essential amino acid methionine. It is a co-factor in three important biochemical pathways, and consequently SAMe is synthesized in cells throughout the body. Because of the important biochemical reactions that it regulates, studies are reporting that SAMe is beneficial for a wide variety of health and medical conditions.

■ SYMPTOMS AND CAUSES OF DEFICIENCY

Normally our bodies produce SAMe from the amino acid methionine. Because vitamin B_{12} and folic acid are necessary for the synthesis of SAMe, a deficiency of these vitamins can lead to a depletion of SAMe. Although no specific condition is associated with a lack of SAMe, problems that likely would develop from a deficiency of SAMe include depression, poor liver detoxification, and elevated homocysteine.

■ BIOLOGICAL FUNCTIONS AND EFFECTS

The functions and effects of SAMe are as follows:

- *Methylation reactions:* SAMe functions as a methyl donor for the synthesis of nucleic acids (DNA and RNA), proteins, phospholipids, catecholamines, and various neurotransmitters.

- *Transsulfuration:* SAMe is the precursor in the sulfur metabolic pathways for the synthesis of cysteine, glutathione, and taurine.

- *Polyamines:* SAMe is necessary for the synthesis of a group of compounds collectively referred to as polyamines, consisting of spermidine, puescine, and spermine. These polyamines are essential for cellular growth and differentiation, gene expression, protein phosphorylation, neuron regeneration, and the repair of DNA.

- *Antioxidant production:* Because SAMe is necessary for the synthesis of the antioxidant glutathione, it plays a role in protecting the body from free radical-induced aging damage.

- *Detoxification:* Glutathione is important for detoxification in the liver. Glutathione depletion usually is found in individuals with liver malfunction. SAMe supplementation promotes the synthesis of glutathione, which improves liver function and detoxification.

- *Healthy cellular membranes:* The ratio between phosphatidylcholine (PC) and cholesterol in cellular membranes determines their relative flexibility or stiffness. PC promotes flexibility, whereas cholesterol promotes stiffness. Because SAMe is an important facilitator of phosphatidyl choline synthesis, it plays a role in promoting more pliant cellular membranes. Stiffer cell membranes are not able to transmit cellular signals as effectively, and it is more difficult for neuropeptides and other messenger molecules to fit into receptor sites when cellular membranes are stiff.

- *Nerve protection:* SAMe protects against neuronal death caused by anoxia (lack of oxygen). It regenerates nerves and promotes remyelination of nerve fibers.

- *Liver protection:* SAMe protects the liver against alcohol, drugs, and cytokines, protects against cholestasis (bile impairment or blockage), and may protect against chronic active hepatitis. It also protects against liver damage caused by MAO inhibitors and anticonvulsants, and it reverses hyperbilirubinaemia.

■ SIDE EFFECTS AND TOXICITY

SAMe has no reported toxicity. A few minor side effects have been occasionally reported, including dry mouth, nausea, and restlessness. Individuals are urged to consult with their physician before combining SAMe with other antidepressants, or with tryptophan or 5-HTP.

■ RDA AND DOSAGE

No RDA has been set for SAMe. Dosages for SAMe range from 200 to 1600 mg daily in divided doses.

The available form is S-adenosyl methionine.

■ FOOD SOURCES

SAMe does not occur in the foods we eat.

SELENIUM

Drugs that deplete selenium		
■ CORTICOSTEROIDS	■ ORAL CONTRACEPTIVES	■ VALPROIC ACID

UNTIL THE LATE 1950S, selenium was thought to be toxic. Although it can be toxic in high doses, selenium now is recognized as one of the most important nutritional trace minerals. Selenium plays important roles in detoxification and antioxidant defense mechanisms in the body. Research has shown that selenium is one of the most powerful anticancer agents ever tested.

■ SYMPTOMS AND CAUSES OF DEFICIENCY

The symptoms of selenium deficiency include destructive changes to the heart and pancreas, sore muscles, increased fragility of red blood cells, and a weakened immune system. Causes are as follows.

- The primary cause of selenium deficiency is insufficient dietary intake resulting from either poor food choices (as in junk foods and fast foods) or eating foods grown in selenium-depleted soils.

- Selenium is not an essential nutrient for plants and, therefore, many farmlands have become increasingly depleted of selenium because farmers see no need to add it to the soil.

• Food processing causes substantial loss of selenium. For example, whole-wheat bread has twice the selenium as white bread, and brown rice has 15 times more selenium than white rice.

• Human breast milk contains six times more selenium than cow's milk. A cow's-milk diet for infants can contribute to low selenium levels and depressed immune systems in infants.

• Protein-calorie malnutrition can lead to selenium deficiency.

• The Keshan district in China had extremely high rates of childhood cardiomyopathies until it was discovered that the soil was deficient in selenium. Nutritional selenium supplementation has solved the problem.

• Increased rates of various types of cancer are associated with low dietary intake of selenium.

■ BIOLOGICAL FUNCTIONS AND EFFECTS

Selenium has many functions in the body. The following is a synopsis.

• Selenium is an indispensable co-factor for glutathione peroxidase, which is one of the most important antioxidant enzymes in the immune system.

• The antioxidant activities of selenium enable it to protect against heart attacks and strokes.

• As an antioxidant, selenium helps to prevent lipid peroxidation and neutralizes destructive hydrogen peroxide. By neutralizing these types of free radicals, selenium works to prevent cancer and cardiovascular disease.

• Selenium is a powerful anticancer nutrient. Numerous epidemiological studies have correlated low dietary selenium intakes with higher rates of cancer.

• Selenium is important to the immune system. It has antiviral activity, increases T-lymphocytes, and enhances natural killer cell activity.

• Selenium is capable of detoxifying heavy metal toxins such as mercury and cadmium.

• Selenium greatly reduces the toxicity of the anticancer drug adriamycin without reducing its antitumor activity.

• Selenium has significant anti-inflammatory properties.

• The enzyme that converts thyroid hormone (T_4) to triiodothyronine (T_3, the active form) is a selenium-dependent enzyme.

• Selenium potentiates the antioxidant activity of vitamin E.

■ SIDE EFFECTS AND TOXICITY

Selenium is a trace mineral that can be toxic. Although deaths from selenium toxicity have been reported in livestock, no deaths have been reported in humans.

Symptoms of selenium toxicity include loss of hair and nails, sores on the skin, nervous system abnormalities, digestive dysfunction, and "garlicky" breath.

■ RDA AND DOSAGE

The RDA for selenium is 70 mcg/day for men and 55 mcg/day for women. Pharmacologic doses in the scientific literature range from 50 mcg to 500 mcg/day. Occasionally, physicians have used much higher doses in cancer therapy and to treat cases of acute inflammation.

Available forms are sodium selenite, selenomethioine, and high-selenium yeast.

■ FOOD SOURCES

Whole grains are the best dietary source of selenium, followed by seafood, garlic, liver, eggs, dairy products, and some vegetables, including cabbage, celery, cucumbers, and radishes. The selenium content of foods is directly dependent on the selenium content of the soil. Foods grown on selenium-deficient soils in many areas of the United States have inadequate selenium content.

SILICON

Drugs that deplete silicon

NO STUDIES THAT REPORT DRUG-INDUCED SILICON DEPLETION HAVE BEEN FOUND.

EVEN THOUGH SILICON is the most abundant mineral on earth, only recently was it discovered to be an essential trace mineral. The largest concentrations of silicon are found in the skin and cartilage, but it also occurs in connective tissue, bone, tendons, lymph nodes, trachea (windpipe), aorta of the heart, and the lungs. Inhalation of silicon from the environment is partially responsible for its high occurrence in lung tissue.

Preliminary studies have shown an age-related decline in the silicon content of the skin, arteries, and thymus. At the same time, concentrations remain relatively stable in the heart, kidneys, muscles, and tendons.

■ Symptoms and Causes of Deficiency

Silicon is so abundant in the environment that outright deficiencies do not exist. The discovery of silicon's role as an essential nutrient is quite recent, though, and very little work has been done regarding its metabolic activity and optimal dosage ranges.

Silicon deficiency might be associated with the development of osteoarthritis and some aspects of cardiovascular disease.

Laboratory animals that are fed silicon-deficient diets have retarded growth and incomplete and deformed skeletal development.

■ Biological Functions and Effects

Cell culture studies and work with chicks suggest that silicon somehow stimulates the production of mucopolysaccharides and collagen. Silicon is an important component of the mucopolysaccharides and collagen of connective tissues. As such, it provides strength, rigidity, and flexibility to bones, teeth, tendons, ligaments, cell walls and membranes, nails, and skin. Silicon aids in building the organic matrix for proper mineralization of bones and teeth.

There is some indication that adequate levels of silicon may be associated with lesser risk for developing atherosclerosis. Silicon also may help to limit or inhibit the absorption of aluminum.

■ Side Effects and Toxicity

Toxicity studies focus on silicosis, an occupational lung disease caused by inhaling silicon dioxide dust. This occurs in mining, sandblasting, and the manufacturing of glass, ceramics, abrasives, and petroleum products. Silicosis is characterized by a degenerative fibrosis of the lung tissue.

■ RDA and Dosage

Nutritional guidelines have not been determined. Daily intake of silicon is variously recommended at 5 to 10 mg/day. The estimated average daily dietary intake of silicon is from 20 to 50 mg/day, so most people apparently are getting sufficient silicon.

■ Food Sources

The best food sources of silicon are rice bran and brown rice. Dietary silicon is available in other unrefined grain products and in high-fiber vegetables. Beer contains a high concentration of easily absorbable silicon.

SODIUM

Drugs that deplete sodium

- ACE INHIBITORS
- ACETAZOLAMIDE
- AMINOGLYCOSIDES
- AMPHOTERICIN B
- ASPIRIN AND SALICYLATES

- CHOLINE MAGNESIUM TRISALICYLATE
- CHOLINE SALICYLATE
- COLCHICINE
- HYDROFLUMETHIAZIDE
- INDAPAMIDE

- LOOP DIURETICS
- SSRIS (INCLUDING ZOLOFT®, PAXIL® AND PROZAC®)
- THIAZIDE DIURETICS

SODIUM is one of the body's three major electrolytes (the other two being potassium and chloride). They exist as fully dissociated ions and are the main particles responsible for osmotic pressure in body fluids. Sodium is the primary extracellular electrolyte in body fluids. The ionic strength of these electrolytes enables them to influence the solubility of proteins and other substances throughout the body.

Most Americans consume enormous amounts of sodium, from 10 to 35 times more than the recommended daily intake, much in the form of common table salt and in processed foods. Dietary sodium is easily absorbed from the intestine, and carried by the blood to the kidneys, where it is either filtered out and returned to the blood or is excreted.

■ SYMPTOMS AND CAUSES OF DEFICIENCY

Sodium deficiency is rare in humans. Conditions that could cause sodium deficiency include starvation, excessive vomiting, severe diarrhea, and excessive perspiration in conjunction with lack of water. Symptoms of sodium deficiency are muscle weakness, poor concentration, memory loss, dehydration, and loss of appetite.

■ BIOLOGICAL FUNCTIONS AND EFFECTS

The major effects of sodium are as follows:

- In regulating body fluids, sodium has a major role in the regulation of blood pressure.

- Sodium ions play a critical role in the transmission of electrochemical impulses for nerve function and muscle contraction.

- Sodium helps regulate the acid/alkaline balance in the blood and lymph fluids.

- Sodium helps to control and operate the sodium/potassium pump. This helps to make the cell walls permeable and facilitates the transport of materials across cell membranes.

- Sodium helps regulate the transport and excretion of carbon dioxide.

■ SIDE EFFECTS AND TOXICITY

High intake of sodium is associated with edema and elevated blood pressure.

■ RDA AND DOSAGE

Sodium has no RDA. A reasonable dietary intake is from 1 to 3 grams per day.

■ FOOD SOURCES

Table salt is the most concentrated source of sodium. Enormous amounts of sodium are used in cooking and food processing. Often this "hidden salt" contributes more to an individual's daily diet than does the salt shaker. Protein foods generally contain more sodium than vegetables and grains. Fruits contain almost no sodium.

SULFUR

Drugs that deplete sulfur

NO STUDIES THAT REPORT DRUG-INDUCED DEPLETION OF SULFUR HAVE BEEN FOUND.

IN THE BODY, sulfur is found primarily as a component of the four sulfur-containing amino acids cystine, cysteine, methionine, and taurine. Although all proteins contain sulfur, it is most prevalent in the keratin of skin and hair and in insulin. Tissues of the joints contain high levels of a sulfur-containing compound called chondroitin sulfate. Two B-vitamins, thiamin and biotin, contain sulfur, as does heparin, which is an anticoagulant synthesized primarily in the liver. Small amounts of sulfur exist in the body as organic sulfates and sulfites.

Sulfur plays an important role in determining the shape, structure, and functionality of proteins. The sulfur-containing amino acids in proteins can create crosslinks by forming disulfide bonds, which act to strengthen and stabilize proteins. Sulfur exists in its reduced form in cysteine and in an oxidized form as a double molecule in cystine.

Sulfur has a characteristic odor. The smell from burning feathers, hair, skin, or nails is from its sulfur content, and "smelly" foods such as onions and garlic contain significant amounts of sulfur.

■ SYMPTOMS AND CAUSES OF DEFICIENCY

Deficiency symptoms related to sulfur are unknown. A diet severely lacking in protein could cause a sulfur deficiency.

■ BIOLOGICAL FUNCTIONS AND EFFECTS

The major role of sulfur, as part of amino acids, is to provide structure to proteins and mucopolysaccharides such as chondroitin sulfate and collagen. Specific functions and effects are as follows:

- Sulfur, through disulfide (–S–S–) or sulfhydryl (–SH) bonds, gives proteins their characteristic different shapes. For example, hair curliness comes from the presence of disulfide bonds of cystine in hair.
- Sulfur plays an important metabolic role as a sulfhydryl group on the active site of coenzyme A.
- Sulfur, in conjunction with magnesium, takes part in the metabolic detoxification of sulfuric acid in the body for excretion in the urine.
- Sulfur-containing lipids (sulfolipids) are found in the liver, kidneys, and brain.
- Sulfur is necessary for all of the biochemical processes involving thiamin, biotin, and lipoic acid.
- The hormone insulin consists of 51 amino acids in 2 polypeptide chains. The two parallel chains are joined by two disulfide bridges.

■ SIDE EFFECTS AND TOXICITY

No toxicity is associated with sulfur. Excesses are efficiently excreted in the urine.

■ RDA AND DOSAGE

No RDA has been set for sulfur. The diet of most Americans is high in protein and provides more than adequate amounts of sulfur.

■ FOOD SOURCES

Protein-rich foods are good sources of sulfur.

VANADIUM

Drugs that deplete vanadium

NO STUDIES THAT REPORT DRUG-INDUCED DEPLETION OF VANADIUM HAVE BEEN FOUND.

HOW ESSENTIAL VANADIUM is in humans has yet to be established with certainty. In the late 1960s it was found to be an essential trace mineral for plant nutrition, and in the early 1970s it was discovered to be an essential nutrient for animals. It probably is essential for humans, too, but some debate still surrounds this issue. Nonetheless, interest in vanadium as a nutritional substance has been building steadily over the past twenty years or so.

Vanadium is a transition metal. As such, it has biochemical properties similar to chromium, molybdenum, manganese, and iron. Vanadium functions primarily as a co-factor, which enhances or inhibits various enzymes.

Vanadium accumulates primarily in organ tissues, with the highest concentrations in the liver, kidneys, and bone. Bone seems to be the long-term storage site for vanadium, and storage of accessible vanadium is primarily in fat and blood lipids.

■ SYMPTOMS AND CAUSES OF DEFICIENCY

No cases of vanadium deficiency are known.

■ BIOLOGICAL FUNCTIONS AND EFFECTS

The most significant research on vanadium to date involves its insulin-like properties and its possible role in treating diabetes. Vanadium and vanadyl salts stimulate glucose metabolism. When given to patients with Type II diabetes, it markedly decreases blood glucose levels.

Vanadium produces its insulin-like effects in the liver by (a) decreasing the activity of the gluconeogenesis enzyme, glucose-6-phosphatase, (b) increasing the activity of two glycolytic enzymes, glucokinase and phosphofructokinase, and (c) increasing the production of glycogen.

In addition:

• Vanadium may have a functional role as a building material in bones and teeth.

• Although the biochemical and physiological roles of vanadium are not yet fully understood, it may be involved in the following processes:

– NADPH oxidation reactions

– lipoprotein lipase activity

– amino acid transport

– the growth of red blood cells.

• At higher dosage levels, vanadium seems to be able to assist in lowering elevated blood cholesterol and triglyceride levels.

• Vanadium is a potent inhibitor of Na^+K^+ ATPase enzymes.

■ SIDE EFFECTS AND TOXICITY

Vanadium has no known toxicity as a dietary nutrient in humans, but it can be absorbed through inhalation, and excessive exposure could be toxic. Vanadium is used as a catalyst in a wide variety of industrial processes, and occasionally, as a result of industrial accidents, vanadium is inhaled to the extent that it becomes toxic.

Experimentally induced vanadium toxicity in animal studies produces reproductive and developmental abnormalities, including decreased fertility, birth defects, and death of the embryo.

■ RDA AND DOSAGE

Dietary requirements for vanadium have not been established. To date, little is known about human nutritional needs for vanadium or whether the amount or type that Americans absorb is adequate. The daily requirement for vanadium is estimated to be about 10 mcg/day. The average American diet contains from 15 to 30 mcg/day, which is more than enough to satisfy nutritional needs.

■ FOOD SOURCES

Fats and vegetable oils are the richest food sources of vanadium. Vanadium also occurs in grains, meats, fish, and nuts. Other foods and spices that contain vanadium are dill seeds, parsley, black pepper, and mushrooms.

VITAMIN A (RETINOL)

Drugs that deplete vitamin A (retinol)

■ CHOLESTYRAMINE	■ CORTICOSTERIODS	■ NEOMYCIN
■ COLESTIPOL	■ MINERAL OIL	

VITAMIN A was the first fat-soluble vitamin to be recognized, in 1913. It was found to prevent night blindness and xerophthalmia. In 1932, beta-carotene (pro-vitamin A) was discovered to be the precursor to vitamin A. Vitamin A is necessary for vision, for the growth and maintenance of epithelial tissues, and for the growth and development of bones. It also regulates immunity and reproduction and has anticancer properties.

• Vitamin A belongs to a class of compounds called retinoids, which occur only in animal products. Retinoids with vitamin A activity are found in nature in three different forms: (a) the alcohol, retinol, (b) the aldehyde, retinal or retinaldehyde, and (c) the acid, retinoic acid.

• Beta-carotene consists of two molecules of vitamin A linked head to head. Enzymes in the intestinal tract split beta-carotene into two molecules of vitamin A whenever the body needs it.

• To be properly absorbed from the digestive tract, vitamin A requires fats as well as minerals.

• Substantial amounts of vitamin A are stored in the liver and, therefore, it does not have to be supplied in the diet daily.

■ SYMPTOMS AND CAUSES OF DEFICIENCY

• Vitamin A deficiency can be caused by inadequate dietary intake or bodily dysfunction that interferes with absorption, storage, or transport of vitamin A.

• Deficiency of vitamin A is associated with the development and promotion of epithelial cell cancers in various glands and organs in the body.

• Night blindness (nyctalopia) is the classic vision problem resulting from vitamin A deficiency. Xerophthalmia (drying and hardening of the membranes that line the eyes) also can develop. This condition causes blindness in hundreds of thousands of infants and children yearly worldwide but seldom occurs in the United States.

• Long-term vitamin A deficiency causes the skin to become dry, scaly, and rough, a condition called keratinization, in which small, hard bumps develop on the skin because hair follicles plug up with a hard protein called keratin.

• Vitamin A deficiency in infants and children hinders their growth and development. Bone deformities and dental problems often result.

■ BIOLOGICAL FUNCTIONS AND EFFECTS

Vitamin A functions in the following ways in the body:

• Vitamin A plays an essential role in vision. It interacts with a photosensitive pigment in the retina that facilitates night vision.

• Vitamin A plays an important role in maintaining the integrity of all epithelial tissue. Many studies show that adequate intake of vitamin A is associated with reduced risk to various epithelial-cell cancers (mouth, skin, lungs, bladder, breast, stomach, cervix).

• By maintaining healthy epithelial cells (surface cells of many glands, organs, and skin), vitamin A helps to create barriers to infections.

• Vitamin A is essential for the growth of bone and soft tissue. It also is necessary for the formation of tooth enamel in the development of teeth.

■ SIDE EFFECTS AND TOXICITY

Because vitamin A is fat-soluble, excesses can accumulate to toxic levels in fatty tissues. Signs of vitamin A toxicity include dry, itchy skin, brittle nails, hair loss, bone pain, gingivitis, headaches, muscle and joint pains, anorexia, fatigue, diarrhea, increased infections, and enlarged liver and abnormal liver function.

Hypervitaminosis A has been reported in adults who have been taking in excess of 50,000 I.U. daily for several years, as well as in a case of taking a water-soluble synthetic vitamin A at 18,500 to 60,000 I.U. for several months.

Doses greater than 10,000 I.U. can be toxic to a fetus. Therefore, women who are pregnant and women of childbearing age who can become pregnant should not take more than 10,000 I.U./day.

■ RDA AND DOSAGE

The RDA for vitamin A is 5,000 I.U./day. No RDA has been set for beta-carotene. Pharmacologic doses in the scientific literature usually range from 10,000 I.U. to 35,000 I.U. Occasional applications can go much higher but should not be attempted without medical supervision.

Dosages of vitamin A and beta-carotene sometimes are measured in terms of retinol equivalents (R.E.). One R.E. (equal to 1 mcg) is equivalent to 5 I.U.

■ FOOD SOURCES

Good food sources of vitamin A are liver, kidney, butter, egg yolk, whole milk and cream, and fortified skim milk. Good food sources of pro-vitamin A (beta-carotene) are yellow and dark green leafy vegetables (carrots, sweet potatoes, squash, collards, spinach) and yellow fruit (apricots, peaches, cantaloupe). Cod liver oil and halibut fish oil contain high levels of vitamin A and have been used therapeutically.

VITAMIN B₁ (THIAMIN)

Drugs that deplete vitamin B₁ (thiamin)

■ AMINOGLYCOSIDES	■ FUROSEMIDE	■ SULFONAMIDES
■ BUMETANIDE	■ MACROLIDES	■ TETRACYCLINES
■ CEPHALOSPORINS	■ ORAL CONTRACEPTIVES	■ TORSEMIDE
■ ETHACRYNIC ACID	■ PENICILLINS	■ TRIMETHOPRIM
■ FLUOROQUINOLONES	■ PHENYTOIN	■ ZONISAMIDE

VITAMIN B₁, also known as thiamin, was the first of the B vitamins to be discovered. It was isolated in 1926 as a water-soluble, crystalline, yellowish-white powder with a salty, slightly nutty taste. In 1936, chemists accomplished the synthesis and determined its chemical formula.

Beriberi is the classic syndrome resulting from a vitamin B₁ deficiency. This disease is more prevalent in Asian countries where polished rice is a dietary staple. When beriberi occurs in the United States, it is seen most commonly in severely malnourished infants and elderly people. In adults, chronic dieting, alcoholism, and diets consisting primarily of highly processed, refined foods are causes of vitamin B₁ deficiency.

■ SYMPTOMS AND CAUSES OF DEFICIENCY

Deficiencies of vitamin B_1 manifest primarily as disorders of the neuro-muscular, intestinal, and cardiovascular systems. Deficiency symptoms include depression, irritability, memory loss, mental confusion, indigestion, weight loss, anorexia, muscular weakness, sore calf muscles, edema, rapid pulse rate, heart palpitation, fatigue, loss of reflexes in the legs, defective muscular coordination, and nerve inflammation including "pins and needles" and numbness.

Insufficiency of thiamin is one of the most common nutritional deficiencies in the United States. One U.S. Department of Agriculture study reported that 45% of Americans consume less than the RDA of thiamin. Vitamin B_1 is easily destroyed or lost during cooking because it is heat-sensitive and water-soluble. Vitamin B_1 also is depleted by diuretic drugs and intestinal conditions such as diarrhea, as well as malabsorption because of lactose intolerance and celiac disease (gliadin or wheat sensitivity).

Alcohol interferes with the absorption of Vitamin B_1, and this vitamin is necessary for the metabolism of alcohol. Severe deficiency associated with alcohol consumption produces a condition called Wernicke–Korsakoff syndrome, with symptoms ranging from mild confusion to severely impaired memory and cognitive function, and coma.

■ BIOLOGICAL FUNCTIONS AND EFFECTS

To be metabolically active, vitamin B_1 must combine with phosphoric acid to form the important coenzyme thiamin pyrophosphate (TPP). Once converted to its active form:

- Thiamin is required by every cell in the body to make ATP, the body's primary fuel and energy source.
- Thiamin plays a major role in converting glucose into biological energy.
- Thiamin is necessary for maintaining nerve tissues, nerve function, and nerve transmissions.
- Thiamin is important in maintaining muscular function, especially of the heart.
- Thiamin is required for the synthesis of acetylcholine, which is the primary neurotransmitter involved in thought and memory processes.
- Thiamin is necessary for the maintenance and proper functioning of muscles, especially heart muscles.
- Thiamin is involved in the synthesis of fatty acids.

■ SYMPTOMS OF TOXICITY

Thiamin is water-soluble, so it is eliminated through the urinary and other body systems rather than being stored in the body. Accumulation to toxic levels is unlikely. Overdose and toxicity would require high doses (in the multiple-gram range).

■ RDA AND DOSAGE

The RDA for vitamin B_1 is 1.5 mg/day. Therapeutic dosage ranges in the scientific literature vary from 10 mg to 100 mg per day in divided doses, although some applications use even larger doses.

■ FOOD SOURCES

All plant and animal foods contain vitamin B_1, although most are only in low concentrations. The richest sources are brewer's yeast and organ meats. Whole-grain cereals comprise the most important dietary source of vitamin B_1 in the typical human diet.

VITAMIN B_2 (RIBOFLAVIN)

Drugs that deplete vitamin B_2 (riboflavin)

- ACETOPHENAZINE
- AMINOGLYCOSIDES
- AMITRIPTYLINE
- AMOXAPINE
- CEPHALOSPORINS
- CHLORPROMAZINE
- CLOMIPRAMINE
- DESIPRAMINE
- DOXEPIN
- FLUOROQUINOLONES
- FLUPHENAZINE
- IMIPRAMINE
- MACROLIDES
- MESORIDAZINE
- METHDILAZINE
- METHOTRIMEPRAZINE
- NORTRIPTYLINE
- ORAL CONTRACEPTIVES
- PENICILLINS
- PERPHENAZINE
- PROCHLORPERAZINE
- PROMAZINE
- PROMETHAZINE
- PROTRIPTYLINE
- SULFONAMIDES
- TETRACYCLINES
- THIORIDAZINE
- TRIFLUOPERAZINE
- TRIMETHOPRIM
- TRIMIPRAMINE

LIKE OTHER B VITAMINS, vitamin B_2 is water-soluble. Because it is not stored in sufficient amounts in the body, it must be supplied daily. Vitamin B_2 is absorbed from the upper part of the small intestine and is absorbed better when taken with food. Only approximately 15% is absorbed if taken alone versus 60% absorption with food. Riboflavin belongs to a group of yellow fluorescent pigments called flavins. In its pure state, riboflavin is a yellow crystalline powder with a slight odor. When excreted, it gives the urine a characteristic bright yellow color.

■ SYMPTOMS AND CAUSES OF DEFICIENCY

Vitamin B_2 deficiencies affect primarily the skin, eyes, and mucous membranes of the intestinal tract. Deficiencies seldom occur alone but, rather, as a component of multiple nutrient deficiencies. Additional symptoms include:

chelosis (cracked corners of the mouth)

inflamed mucous membranes

soreness and burning of the lips, mouth, and tongue (possibly magenta-colored tongue)

reddening, tearing, burning, and itching of the eyes

eyes tiring easily

eyes highly sensitive to light

dry, itchy, scaly skin (seborrheic dermatitis)

scaling eczema of the face and genitals.

In severe long-term deficiency, damage to nerve tissue can cause depression and hysteria. Riboflavin is heat-stable but sensitive to destruction by light. Because it is water-soluble, substantial amounts are lost by leaching into water when cooking. The vitamin exists in the germ and bran of grains, so milling and processing of grains result in substantial losses.

Individuals at greatest risk for riboflavin deficiency are alcoholics, infants, and elderly people who have unbalanced, nutritionally deficient diets.

■ BIOLOGICAL FUNCTIONS AND EFFECTS

Riboflavin has the following functions and effects:

• Riboflavin facilitates the metabolism of carbohydrates, fats, and proteins.

• Combined with phosphoric acid, riboflavin becomes part of two important flavin co-enzymes, FMN (flavin mononucleotide) and FAD (flavin adenine dinucleotide). FMN and FAD are known to bind to more than 100 flavoprotein enzymes, which catalyze oxidation-reduction reactions in cells. These enzymes include the oxidases, which function aerobically, and dehydrogenases, which function anaerobically.

• Riboflavin plays a vital role in converting carbohydrates to ATP in the production of energy. In energy production, flavoprotein enzymes function as hydrogen carriers in the electron transport system, resulting in the production of energy within the mitochondria.

• Riboflavin contributes important antioxidant activity, both by itself and as part of the enzyme glutathione reductase.

• Riboflavin is necessary for growth and reproduction.

• Riboflavin is essential to the healthy growth of skin, hair, and nails.

■ SYMPTOMS OF TOXICITY

There is no known toxicity for riboflavin. Its negligible storage and easy excretion make it a safe nutrient.

■ RDA AND DOSAGE

A survey by the U.S. Department of Agriculture estimated that 34% of Americans get less than the RDA of vitamin B_2 daily.[11] The RDA for vitamin B_2 is 1.7 mg/day. Pregnant women, nursing mothers, and individuals who exercise heavily require somewhat higher intakes.

High-potency vitamin formulations and therapeutic dosages are in the range of 15 mg to 50 mg daily in divided doses.

■ FOOD SOURCES

The best sources of vitamin B_2 are liver, milk, and dairy products. Moderate sources include meats, dark green vegetables, eggs, avocados, oysters, mushrooms, and fish (especially salmon and tuna).

VITAMIN B₃ (NIACIN)

Drugs that deplete vitamin B₃ (niacin)

- AMINGLYCOSIDES
- CEPHALOSPORINS
- CYCLOSERINE
- ESTROGENS, CONJUGATED
- ESTROGENS, ESTERIFIED
- FLUOROQUINOLONES
- ISONIAZID
- MACROLIDES
- ORAL CONTRACEPTIVES
- PENICILLINS
- SULFONAMIDES
- TETRACYCLINES
- TRIMETHOPRIM

NIACIN is a water-soluble B-vitamin that functions metabolically as a component of two important coenzymes: nicotinamide adenine dinucleotide (NAD) and nicotinamide adenine dinucleotide phosphate (NADP), known as the pyridine nucleotides.

■ SYMPTOMS AND CAUSES OF DEFICIENCY

Severe deficiency of niacin is known as pellagra, which means "rough skin." Symptoms of pellagra are the "3 Ds": dermatitis, dementia, and diarrhea. Pellagra occurs in areas where nutrition is meager and corn is the dietary staple (tryptophan and niacin are poorly absorbed from corn.) In Mexico, however, where corn is treated with lye before use, deficiency is less common because the alkali increases absorption of tryptophan.

The parts of the body most affected by niacin deficiency are:

• *Skin:* cracked, pigmented, scaly dermatitis, especially on parts exposed to the sun.

• *Intestinal tract:* inflammation of mucous membranes, causing many digestive abnormalities including swollen tongue and diarrhea.

• *Nervous system:* mental confusion and disorientation leading to psychosis or delirium.

■ BIOLOGICAL FUNCTIONS AND EFFECTS

Niacin-containing coenzymes NAD and NADP are involved in more than 200 reactions in the metabolism of carbohydrates, fatty acids, and amino acids, making it vital in supplying energy to, and maintaining the function of, every cell in the body. Specific functions of niacin and its forms are summarized in the following:

- Niacin is especially important in the oxidation-reduction reactions in the Krebs cycle, involving the production of energy from carbohydrates.

- Niacin is useful in treating elevated blood cholesterol levels: It reduces LDL ("bad") cholesterol and triglycerides and increases HDL ("good") cholesterol.

  In one study, niacin reduced the recurrence rate of heart attacks by nearly 30% at dosages of about 2 grams per day and provided a 11% reduction in the overall mortality rate.[12]

- Niacinamide has been shown to have anti-anxiety benefit resembling benzodiazepines, and Italian doctors report using it successfully to help addicted patients withdraw from benzodiazepines.

- Doses of nicotinic acid in the 75 mg range stimulate the release of histamines, which causes temporary vasodilation and the characteristic "niacin flush."

- Niacin has been identified as part of the glucose tolerance factor of yeast, which enhances the response to insulin.

■ SYMPTOMS OF TOXICITY

Large doses of niacin cause transient side effects such as tingling sensations, flushing of the skin, and head throbbing because of its vasodilating action. These effects disappear within 20 to 30 minutes.

The sustained-release form of niacin can be toxic to the liver and should not be used.

■ RDA AND DOSAGE

The RDA for adult males is 18 mg/day and for adult females is 13 mg/day. Therapeutic dosage ranges in the scientific literature vary from 30 mg to 2,000 mg per day. In some studies, however, dosages up to 6 grams per day have been used. Dosages above 2 grams per day should be administered only under medical supervision.

Available forms are nicotinic acid (niacin), niacinamide (nicotinamide), and inositol hexaniacinate.

■ FOOD SOURCES

Both niacin and its precursor, tryptophan, are included when determining the niacin content of foods. Lean meats, poultry, fish, and peanuts are good sources of both niacin and tryptophan. The best sources of niacin are organ meats, brewer's yeast, milk, legumes, peanuts and peanut butter. Intestinal bacteria also synthesize niacin.

VITAMIN B$_5$ (PANTOTHENIC ACID)

Drugs that deplete vitamin B$_5$ (pantothenic acid)

- ASPIRIN AND SALICYLATES

D R. ROGER WILLIAMS discovered vitamin B$_5$ in 1933. Because it is present in all cells, he named it pantothenic acid, from the Greek word "panthothen," meaning "everywhere." Pantothenic acid is necessary for the production of some hormones and neurotransmitters, and it is involved in the metabolism of all carbohydrates, fats, and proteins.

Vitamin B$_5$ is most commonly available commercially as calcium pantothenate. After absorption, pantothenic acid is first converted to a sulfur-containing compound called pantotheine. Pantotheine then is converted into coenzyme A, the only known biologically active form of pantothenic acid.

■ SYMPTOMS AND CAUSES OF DEFICIENCY

Pantothenic acid is so widely available in foods that a deficiency in humans is virtually unknown. Experimentally induced deficiencies manifest as problems related to the skin, liver, thymus, and nerves.

■ BIOLOGICAL FUNCTIONS AND EFFECTS

As a constituent of coenzyme A (CoA), pantothenic acid participates in a wide variety of enzymatic reactions within cells throughout the body. CoA is involved in the release of energy from carbohydrates in the Krebs cycle. Pantothenic acid can provide an anti-stress effect because CoA is necessary for the synthesis of steroid hormones and proper functioning of the adrenal glands. CoA functions in the production of fats, cholesterol, and bile acids.

Other functions and effects of pantothenic acid are the following:

• Pantothenic acid is necessary for the synthesis of acetylcholine, phospholipids, and porphyrin in the hemoglobin of red blood cells.

• Pantothenic acid may help to boost energy and athletic ability because of its role in the metabolism of carbohydrates.

• Pantothenic acid helps to detoxify alcohol by participating in the metabolism of acetaldehyde.

- Pantothenic acid has been reported to improve the stress reactions of well nourished individuals and to relieve "burning feet" syndrome.

■ SYMPTOMS OF TOXICITY

No known toxic effects arise from taking large doses of pantothenic acid. Ingestion of large amounts of pantothenic acid may cause diarrhea.

■ RDA AND DOSAGE

The RDA for pantothenic acid is 10 mg per day. Pharmacologic doses in the scientific literature range from 50 mg to 1000 mg per day.

Available forms are calcium pantothenate and dexpanthenol.

■ FOOD SOURCES

Pantothenic acid is present in all plant and animal tissues. Best sources of this vitamin include eggs, liver, fish, chicken, whole-grain breads and cereals, and legumes. Other good sources are cauliflower, broccoli, lean beef, white and sweet potatoes, and tomatoes.

VITAMIN B$_6$ (PYRIDOXINE)

Drugs that deplete vitamin B$_6$ (pyridoxine)

■ AMINOGLYCOSIDES	■ FLUOROQUINOLONES	■ PHENELZINE
■ BUMETANIDE	■ FUROSEMIDE	■ PHENOBARBITAL
■ CEPHALOSPORINS	■ HYDRALAZINE	■ QUINESTROL
■ DIETHYLSTILBESTEROL	■ ISONIAZID	■ SULFONAMIDES
■ ESTROGENS, CONJUGATED	■ LEVODOPA	■ TETRACYCLINES
	■ MACROLIDES	■ THEOPHYLLINE
■ ESTROGENS, ESTERIFIED	■ ORAL CONTRACEPTIVES	■ TORSEMIDE
	■ PENICILLAMINE	■ TRIMETHOPRIM
■ ETHACRYNIC ACID	■ PENICILLINS	

VITAMIN B$_6$ is necessary for the proper functioning of more than 60 enzymes. Many of its activities are related to the metabolism of amino acids and other protein-related compounds such as hemoglobin, serotonin, various hormones, and the prostaglandins. After entering a cell, vitamin B$_6$ is phosphorylated, which converts it into its active form, pyridoxal phosphate (PLP).

■ SYMPTOMS AND CAUSES OF DEFICIENCY

Deficiencies of vitamin B$_6$ manifest primarily as dermatologic, circulatory, and neurologic changes. Because of its many metabolic roles, pyridoxine also produces a wide variety of deficiency symptoms. These include:

depression

sleep disturbances

nerve inflammation

PMS

lethargy

decreased alertness

anemia

altered mobility

elevated homocysteine levels

nausea

vomiting

seborrheic dermatitis

The following B_6 deficiency conditions are explained in greater detail.

• *Depression from inhibition of serotonin synthesis:* Vitamin B_6 is essential for 5-hydroxytryptophan decarboxylase, an enzyme that catalyzes one of the steps in the conversion of tryptophan to serotonin. Thus, a vitamin B_6 deficiency can limit the brain's ability to synthesize serotonin. Low serotonin levels are associated with depression.

• *Insomnia from inhibition of melatonin synthesis:* Melatonin, which is our biochemical sleep trigger, is synthesized from serotonin in the brain. If a vitamin B_6 deficiency inhibits serotonin synthesis, there will be a corresponding decrease in the body's ability to synthesize melatonin, which may cause insomnia.

• *Elevated homocysteine:* Elevated homocysteine now is recognized as one of the most critical independent risk factors for cardiovascular disease. Homocysteine is a toxic intermediate metabolite in the metabolism of the amino acid methionine. It is capable of directly damaging the vascular system and initiating the process of atherosclerosis. Vitamin B_6 is one of the nutrients required to metabolize homocysteine so it doesn't build up in the blood and begin to damage the lining of the blood vessels.

• *PMS:* Vitamin B_6 seems to influence estrogen-induced gene expression. A B_6 deficiency results in a substantial increase in estrogen gene expression. Under these conditions, excess estrogen may be produced, which could cause symptoms such as heavy menstrual flow, tender breasts, irregular bleeding, and emotional mood swings.

In addition to the listed drugs that deplete vitamin B_6, numerous substances in the environment antagonize vitamin B_6. These include alcohol, tobacco smoke, yellow dye #5 (tartrazine), PCBs, rancid fats in fried foods, and the chemical used to accelerate the ripening process of fruits. Because vitamin B_6 is water-soluble, substantial amounts are lost in cooking and food processing.

■ BIOLOGICAL FUNCTIONS AND EFFECTS

Many pyridoxal phosphate enzymes are involved with amino acid metabolism, including: transamination (transfer of amino groups), deamination (removal of amino groups), desulfuration (transfer of sulfhydro groups), and decarboxylation (removal of COOH groups). Additional functions are as follows:

- Vitamin B_6 is necessary for the formation of hemoglobin and the growth of red blood cells.
- Vitamin B_6 is essential for the synthesis of tryptophan, and the conversion of tryptophan to niacin.
- Vitamin B_6 is required for the production of neurotransmitters derived from amino acids such as serotonin, GABA, norepinephrine, acetylcholine, and histamine.
- Vitamin B_6 facilitates conversion of glycogen to glucose for energy production.

Vitamin B_6 supplementation has the following effects:

- Vitamin B_6 is useful in treating depression. Vitamin B_6 is involved in the synthesis of serotonin, which elevates mood.
- Vitamin B_6 is useful in treating premenstrual syndrome (PMS) associated with oral contraceptives (estrogens inhibit the absorption of vitamin B_6).
- Vitamin B_6 may be beneficial in preventing and treating repetitive motion injuries such as carpal tunnel syndrome.
- Vitamin B_6 helps to prevent atherosclerosis by metabolizing homocysteine.

Some individuals with arthritis respond to pyridoxine. Because it is safe to use, it might be worth trying in all patients with arthritis. Many autistic infants respond to vitamin B_6.

■ SYMPTOMS OF TOXICITY

Vitamin B_6 can be toxic to the nerves when taken in large doses. Several cases have been reported in people taking 2 grams or more per day. Symptoms included tingling in the hands and feet, decreased muscle coordination, and a stumbling gait. All recovered without problems.

■ RDA AND DOSAGE

Vitamin B_6 is one of the most commonly deficient nutrients in the United States. One study by the U.S. Department of Agriculture study reported that approximately 80% of Americans consumed less than the RDA for vitamin B_6, which is 2 mg/day. Therapeutic dosage ranges in the scientific literature vary from 10 mg to 100 mg per day, although some applications go higher. Available forms are pyridoxine hydrochloride, pyridoxal hydrochloride, and pyridoxal-5'-phosphate.

■ FOOD SOURCES

The best sources of pyridoxine are brewer's yeast, wheat germ, organ meats (especially liver), peanuts, legumes, potatoes, and bananas. The beneficial intestinal bacteria synthesize Vitamin B_6.

VITAMIN B_{12} (CYANOCOBALAMIN)

Drugs that deplete vitamin B_{12} (cyanocobalamin)

- AMINOGLYCOSIDES
- CEPHALOSPORINS
- CHLOROTRIANISENE
- CHOLESTYRAMINE
- CIMETIDINE
- CLOFIBRATE
- COLCHICINE
- COLESTIPOL
- CO-TRIMOXAZOLE
- FAMOTIDINE

- FLUOROQUINOLONES
- LANSOPRAZOLE
- MACROLIDES
- METFORMIN
- NEOMYCIN
- NEVIRAPINE
- NIZATIDINE
- OMEPRAZOLE
- ORAL CONTRACEPTIVES

- PENICILLINS
- PHENYTOIN
- POTASSIUM CHLORIDE
  (TIMED-RELEASE)
- RANITIDINE
- SULFONAMIDES
- TETRACYCLINES
- TRIMETHOPRIM
- ZIDOVUDINE

VITAMIN B_{12} was isolated from liver extract in 1948 and has been shown to control pernicious anemia. Cobalamin is the generic name for vitamin B_{12}, because it contains the heavy metal cobalt. Vitamin B_{12} is an essential growth factor and plays a vital role in the metabolism of all cells, especially those of the intestinal tract, bone marrow, and nervous tissue.

Several different cobalamin compounds exhibit vitamin B_{12} activity. Cyanocobalamin, the most stable and most active form of the vitamin, contains a cyanide group that is well below toxic levels and is totally safe. Vitamin B_{12} is a water-soluble, red crystalline substance. Its red color comes from the presence of cobalt in the molecule.

A protein in gastric secretions called intrinsic factor binds to vitamin B_{12} and facilitates its absorption. Without intrinsic factor, less than 1% of vitamin B_{12} is absorbed. Relatively large amounts of vitamin B_{12} can be stored in the liver.

■ SYMPTOMS AND CAUSES OF DEFICIENCY

Vitamin B_{12} deficiencies manifest primarily as anemia and neurologic changes. Vitamin B_{12} deficiency inhibits the synthesis of DNA, which affects the growth and repair of all cells. Symptoms of vitamin B_{12} deficiency include fatigue, peripheral neuropathy, tongue and mouth irregularities, macrocytic anemia (abnormally enlarged red blood cells), depression, confusion and memory loss (especially in the elderly), poor blood clotting and easy bruising, dermatitis and skin sensitivity, loss of appetite, nausea, and vomiting.

Anemia is the first symptom of vitamin B_{12} deficiency. Pernicious anemia results from either inadequate vitamin B_{12} intake or reduced gastric (stomach) secretion of intrinsic factor, which reduces the absorption of B_{12}.

Elderly people are most susceptible to vitamin B_{12} deficiency because their stomach cells lose the ability to produce intrinsic factor, which is necessary for B_{12} absorption. Deficiencies in elderly people often cause varying degrees of neuropsychiatric symptoms such as moodiness, confusion, abnormal gait, memory loss, agitation, delusions, dizziness, dementia, and hallucinations.

Meatless diets are deficient in vitamin B_{12}. Therefore, strict vegetarians are urged to use a vitamin B_{12} supplement.

Many drugs inhibit vitamin B_{12} absorption and, when taken over time, can lead to nutrient depletion.

■ BIOLOGICAL FUNCTIONS AND EFFECTS

Cobalamin coenzymes are necessary for converting RNA to DNA. This means that B_{12} plays a central role in replicating the genetic code and makes it a critical growth factor in all cells of the body. Further:

- Vitamin B_{12} is required for the synthesis of myelin, which insulates the nerves and thus is essential to the functioning and maintenance of the nervous system.

- Vitamin B_{12} aids in the synthesis of methionine and in the metabolism of folic acid.

- Vitamin B_{12} is necessary for the maturation of red blood cells.

- Vitamin B_{12} is involved in various aspects of protein, fat, and carbohydrate metabolism.

- Vitamin B_{12} may help to prevent smokers from developing mouth and throat cancer.

- Many asthmatics are helped by vitamin B_{12} therapy.

■ SYMPTOMS OF TOXICITY

There are no known symptoms of toxicity for vitamin B_{12}, even at doses 1000 times greater than the RDA.

■ RDA AND DOSAGE

The RDA for vitamin B_{12} is 6 mcg (micrograms). Pharmacologic dosages in the scientific literature range from 100 mcg up to 2000 mcg.

Intramuscular injection is the most effective route of administration, especially for the elderly. Studies now indicate that oral and sublingual B_{12} is more effectively absorbed than previously thought.

Available forms are cyanocobalamin and methylcobalamin.

■ FOOD SOURCES

Animal protein products supply B_{12}, of which organ meats are the best source, followed by clams, oysters, beef, eggs, milk, chicken, and cheese. Vitamin B_{12} does not occur in fruits, vegetables, grain, or legumes.

VITAMIN C (ASCORBIC ACID)

Drugs that deplete vitamin C (ascorbic acid)

- ASPIRIN
- BUMETANIDE
- CHOLINE MAGNESIUM TRISALICYLATE
- CHOLINE SALICYLATE
- CORTICOSTEROIDS
- ETHACRYNIC ACID
- FUROSEMIDE
- INDOMETHACIN
- ORAL CONTRACEPTIVES
- TETRACYCLINES
- TORSEMIDE

VITAMIN C is the cure for the world's oldest known nutritional deficiency disease, scurvy. In fact, its name is derived from Latin (*a* = not, *scorbutus* = scurvy, meaning without scurvy). Vitamin C was first isolated by Albert Szent–Gyorgyi in 1928 from the adrenal glands of pigs, and was called hexuronic acid. In 1933 it was successfully synthesized, and the name was changed to ascorbic acid.

In his 1972 book *The Healing Factor: Vitamin C Against Disease*, Irwin Stone, M.D., discussed more than 500 studies that reported the value of high doses of vitamin C in preventing and treating about 100 diseases. Research since then has continued to support the vast importance of this nutrient.

Vitamin C is water-soluble and is easily absorbed from the small intestine. Although it is concentrated in many tissues throughout the body, the adrenal glands contain the highest concentration.

Humans are one of the few species that cannot manufacture vitamin C and must depend on the diet, or nutritional supplements, as the source of this vitamin. Vitamin C exists in nature in both its reduced form, L-ascorbic acid, and in its oxidized form, L-dehydroascorbic acid. L-ascorbic acid is the most active form, but they convert to each other back and forth in a reversible equilibrium, and both are antiscorbutic.

■ Symptoms and Causes of Deficiency

Although scurvy is rare in the United States, subclinical vitamin C deficiencies are common. Deficiency symptoms include capillary fragility, hemorrhage, muscular weakness, easy bruising, gums that bleed easily, poor healing of wounds, anemia, poor appetite and growth, and tender and swollen joints.

Causes of deficiency are as follows.

• Stressful situations (both physical and emotional) tend to deplete the body's stores of vitamin C quickly.

• Individuals most likely to have deficiencies include elderly people on poor diets, alcoholics, people who are severely ill or under chronic stress, and infants who are fed only cow's milk.

• Studies have shown that:

– up to 95% of institutionalized elderly people are deficient in vitamin C.

– 75% of cancer patients are deficient in vitamin C.

– 20% of healthy elderly people are deficient in vitamin C.

■ Biological Functions and Effects

Vitamin C is involved in numerous body functions including oxidation-reduction reactions, energy production, metabolism of tyrosine, reduction and storage of iron, and activation of folic acid. Vitamin C is essential in the formation or synthesis of collagen, serotonin, norepinephrine, thyroxine, and some of the corticosteroids. To summarize:

• Vitamin C plays a major role in the synthesis of collagen and elastin (the major structural components of skin), tendons, bone matrix, tooth dentin, blood vessels, and connective tissues between cells. Collectively, collagen is the most abundant protein in the body, comprising 25% to 30% of total body protein.

• Vitamin C is one of the body's most powerful antioxidants. Being water-soluble, it protects all body fluids, within every cell in the body, and is highly concentrated in the brain to protect against brain aging.

• Vitamin C helps the body handle all types of stress. It is required for the synthesis of the body's main stress response hormones in the adrenal glands, including adrenalin, noradrenalin, cortisol, and histamine. Stresses, such as fever, burns, exposure to cold, physical trauma, fractures, high altitude, and radiation, all require larger doses of vitamin C.

• Vitamin C prevents the formation of nitrosamines and dramatically reduces cervical dysplasia, as well as intestinal and cervical cancers. Vitamin C is claimed to prevent formation of bladder tumors, inhibit hyaluronidase (an enzyme found in malignant tumors), slow the degradation of cellular tissue and decrease the invasion of cancerous growth, stimulate production of white blood cells that engulf and destroy cancer cells, and prevent damage from free radicals, which can cause cancer.

• In preventing cardiovascular disease, vitamin C

- increases HDL (good) cholesterol.
- decreases elevated LDL and total cholesterol by conversion to bile acids for excretion.
- is necessary for synthesis of collagen and elastin, which maintain strength and elasticity of blood vessels.
- decreases free radical oxidation of cholesterol.
- decreases levels of lipoprotein(a) or Lp(a), which are known to produce atherosclerosis.

• Plaque in the arteries is an insoluble complex made up of calcium-phospholipid-cholesterol. Sodium ascorbate can convert insoluble plaque to sodium calcium-phospholipid-cholesterol, which is soluble. This conversion helps to reduce atherosclerotic plaque build-up.

• Vitamin C boosts immunity by:

- increasing production of disease-fighting white blood cells (neutrophils, lymphocytes, and natural killer cells).
- increasing levels of the antibodies that fight infections
- increasing the body's production of interferon
- modulating prostaglandin synthesis

• Vitamin C functions as an antihistamine, and as a phosphodiesterase inhibitor (the same action as some asthma medications). Vitamin C reduces the frequency and intensity of bronchial spasms in individuals who have asthma.

• Ascorbic acid is effective in treating most viruses (if enough is used) including herpes, shingles, viral hepatitis, and polio, by stimulating the production of interferons.

• An analysis of 14 placebo-controlled trials shows a 35% average reduction in the duration of the common cold when treated with vitamin C, and a decrease in the severity of symptoms.[13]

• Vitamin C increases the healing of scars, broken bones, burns, and other conditions.

• Vitamin C detoxifies heavy metal toxins such as mercury, lead, cadmium, and nickel.

• Vitamin C is capable of regenerating the antioxidant form of vitamin E.

■ SIDE EFFECTS AND TOXICITY

Vitamin C is nontoxic, and excesses are excreted in the urine. The only significant side effect of an overdose of vitamin C is diarrhea. Approximately 15% of people taking moderately high doses of vitamin C experience abdominal gas, bloating, and cramping. The mineral ascorbates, such as calcium or magnesium ascorbate, are much less acidic and usually solve this problem.

Although vitamin C has not been proven to cause kidney stones, in some individuals its metabolic pathway produces a high amount of oxalic acid, which could be a problem. Therefore, people with a history of gout, kidney stones, or kidney disease should not take high dosages of vitamin C without medical supervision.

Contrary to a common misperception, vitamin C does not destroy vitamin B_{12} and cause pernicious anemia.

Large doses of vitamin C will interfere with tests to determine occult blood in the stool and tests to monitor blood glucose levels in diabetics.

■ RDA AND DOSAGE

The RDA for vitamin C is 60 mg per day. Pharmacologic doses in the scientific literature range from 500 mg up to 20 grams daily. Higher doses of vitamin C should be taken in three or four divided doses throughout the day. Any kind of physical or emotional stress calls for higher intake of vitamin C.

Taking vitamin C to bowel tolerance (just below the diarrhea point) is a therapeutic technique that has gained some acceptance. The intake necessary to reach bowel tolerance varies from person to person.

Available forms are ascorbic acid, calcium ascorbate, magnesium ascorbate, sodium ascorbate, ester C, and ascorbyl palmitate

■ FOOD SOURCES

Food sources for vitamin C are fresh fruits, especially citrus fruits, strawberries, cantaloupe, and currants; and fresh vegetables, especially Brussels sprouts, collard greens, lettuce, cabbage, peas, and asparagus.

VITAMIN D (CALCIFEROL)

Drugs that deplete vitamin D (calciferol)

■ BARBITURATES	■ CORTICOSTEROIDS	■ NIZATIDINE
■ CARBAMAZEPINE	■ FAMOTIDINE	■ PHENOBARTIBAL
■ CHOLESTYRAMINE	■ FOSPHENYTOIN	■ PHENYTOIN
■ CIMETIDINE	■ ISONIAZID	■ RANITIDINE
■ COLESTIPOL	■ MINERAL OIL	■ RIFAMPIN

VITAMIN D was isolated in 1930 and named calciferol. Since then, more metabolites have been found, and the two major forms of this vitamin are now known to be vitamin D_2 (ergocalciferol) and vitamin D_3 (cholecalciferol). Vitamin D is actually a hormone precursor, which the body can manufacture. Therefore, in a classic sense, it is not actually an essential nutrient. Because rickets is related to vitamin D deficiency, however, vitamin D has been traditionally classified as a vitamin.

Vitamin D is known as the "sunshine vitamin." It is formed in the body by the action of the sun's ultraviolet rays on the skin, converting the biological precursor into vitamin D. Vitamin D is a fat-soluble nutrient that is stored in body fats, principally the liver.

■ SYMPTOMS AND CAUSES OF DEFICIENCY

Rickets is the classic childhood vitamin D deficiency disease. Insufficient vitamin D limits calcium absorption, which can produce bones that are not strong enough to withstand the ordinary stresses and strains of weight-bearing. In adults, vitamin D deficiency can result in osteomalacia and osteoporosis. Symptoms of vitamin D deficiency include the following:

• *In children:* knock-knees, bowed legs, spinal curvature, pigeon breast, disfiguring of the skull, and tooth decay and dental problems.

• *In adults:* rheumatic pains, muscle weakness, increased likelihood of fractures of the hip and pelvis, gradual loss of hearing.

Causes of Vitamin D deficiency include inadequate dietary intake; limited exposure to sunlight, which reduces the body's synthesis of vitamin D; and kidney or liver malfunctions that inhibit the conversion of vitamin D to its metabolically active forms.

Vitamin D deficiency increases the risk for osteoporosis by reducing bone mass and bone density. There is no evidence, however, that vitamin D supplementation is effective in treating osteoporosis. Osteomalacia is the adult equivalent of rickets, in which vitamin D deficiency causes softening of the bones, which can lead to deformities. This condition occurs more frequently in elderly people. It can cause rheumatic pain and muscle weakness and increases the likelihood of fractures of the hip and pelvis.

Vitamin D deficiency can cause a gradual hearing loss because demineralization of the bones in the middle ear inhibits the transmission of vibrations to the nerves that communicate with the brain. An additional problem resulting from vitamin D deficiency is phosphorus retention in the kidneys.

■ BIOLOGICAL FUNCTIONS AND EFFECTS

Vitamin D promotes the absorption of calcium and phosphorus for the growth of bones and teeth. For this reason, it is an essential growth nutrient for infants and children. The active form of vitamin D is called calcitrol. Because calcitrol is produced in the kidneys and functions elsewhere in the body as well, it is considered a hormone, with the intestines and bone as its targets. Calcitrol is the most active form of vitamin D, acting in the intestines to promote absorption of calcium and phosphorus. A synopsis of these functions and effects is as follows:

- Vitamin D is involved in the formation (mineralization) of bone, as well as in the mobilization (demineralization) of bone mineral.
- Vitamin D might be helpful in preventing and treating some cancers. Geographical areas with the least amount of sunlight have the highest rates of colorectal and breast cancers. The active form of vitamin D, calcitrol, inhibits the growth of melanoma, leukemia, and breast, lymphoma, and colon cancer cells.
- Calcitrol regulates serum levels of calcium and phosphorus.
- Vitamin D may help to prevent osteoporosis, as it facilitates absorption of calcium from the intestines. Low calcium levels stimulate the parathyroid gland, which initiates pulling calcium out of the bone.
- Some individuals with psoriasis respond to therapy with the active form of vitamin D. Sunlight and ultraviolet light are also often helpful for psoriasis.
- The active form of vitamin D enhances the immune system by stimulating the activity of macrophages.

■ SIDE EFFECTS AND TOXICITY

Vitamin D can be toxic. Excessive intake of this nutrient causes hypercalcemia, calcium deposits in soft tissues such as kidneys, arteries, heart, ear, and lungs. Signs of vitamin D toxicity include headache, weakness, nausea and vomiting, and constipation.

■ RDA AND DOSAGE

The RDA for vitamin D is 400 I.U. per day. Pharmacologic doses in the scientific literature range from 400 I.U. up to 1,000 I.U. daily.

VITAMIN E (ALPHA TOCOPHEROL)

Drugs that deplete vitamin E (alpha tocopherol)

- CHOLESTYRAMINE
- CLOFIBRATE
- COLESTIPOL
- FENOFIBRATE
- GEMFIBROZIL
- HALOPERIDOL
- MINERAL OIL

IN 1932 SCIENTISTS from the University of California-Berkeley discovered a compound in vegetable oils that is necessary for reproduction in rats, and they named it vitamin E.[14] They called it the "anti-sterility vitamin," which turned out to be an unfortunate designation, as it subsequently was found not to cause this result in humans. The same researchers isolated the pure substance from wheat germ oil in 1936 and gave it the chemical name of tocopherol (after the Greek word "tokos," meaning "offspring," and "phero," meaning "to bring forth").

Vitamin E actually is a group of eight compounds including four tocopherols (alpha, beta, gamma, and delta) and four additional tocotrienol derivatives. Alpha tocopherol is the most common and most potent form and is what usually is meant by the term vitamin E. Pure vitamin E compounds are easily oxidized, so they are manufactured as acetate or succinate esters.

Natural vitamin E is d-alpha tocopherol, whereas synthetically produced vitamin E is a mixture consisting of both the d- and l-isomers as dl-alpha tocopherol. Different studies report that natural vitamin E has from 34% to 50% greater bioavailability than synthetic vitamin E.

■ SYMPTOMS AND CAUSES OF DEFICIENCY

Vitamin E is destroyed by heat and oxidation during cooking and food processing. Therefore, reliance on processed foods and fast foods can contribute to depletion of vitamin E. Low levels of selenium and a high intake of polyunsaturated fatty acids both contribute to depletion of vitamin E.

Symptoms of vitamin E deficiency include dry skin, dull dry hair, rupturing of red blood cells resulting in anemia, easy bruising, PMS, fibrocystic breasts, hot flashes, eczema, psoriasis, cataracts, benign prostatic hyperplasia (BPH), poor wound-healing, muscle weakness, and sterility.

Premature infants are likely to be deficient in vitamin E because very little vitamin E is transferred across the placenta from mother to fetus. Breast milk, however, contains enough vitamin E to meet the infant's needs.

■ BIOLOGICAL FUNCTIONS AND EFFECTS

Vitamin E is the body's most important fat-soluble antioxidant. As such, it ensures the stability and integrity of cellular tissues and membranes throughout the body by preventing free radical damage.

Vitamin E (100 I.U./day) causes up to a 40% reduction in the risk to the nation's number-one killer, cardiovascular disease. It accomplishes this by decreasing platelet stickiness, protecting blood vessels against developing atherosclerotic lesions, and protecting LDL-cholesterol against oxidation.

Low levels of vitamin E are associated with greater risk for developing various forms of cancer, including lung, oral, colon, rectal, cervical, pancreatic, and liver. This also may be because of the protective function of vitamin E against free radical damage. In most cases, however, the amount necessary to protect against cancer is substantially greater than the amount provided in the average American diet.

Vitamin E and vitamin E supplementation has the following effects:

• Vitamin E supplementation has been shown to enhance immune system function and increase resistance to infection.

• During heavy exercise, vitamin E markedly reduces the amount of exercise-induced free radical damage to the blood and tissues and also decreases the incidence of exercise-induced injury to muscles.

• Vitamin E protects the eyes against cataracts and macular degeneration.

• Some studies have shown that vitamin E supplementation (from 150 I.U. to 600 I.U. daily) helps many women alleviate the symptoms of PMS.

■ SIDE EFFECTS AND TOXICITY

Although it is fat-soluble, vitamin E is a relatively nontoxic nutrient. Approximately 60% to 70% of the daily dose is excreted in the feces.

Vitamin E can increase blood-clotting time and, therefore, high-level supplementation is not advised without medical supervision for individuals who are taking anticoagulant drugs.

Most individuals studied while taking large doses of vitamin E have not shown toxic effects, but symptoms have been reported from isolated cases in which people were taking more than 1000 I.U. daily, including headache, fatigue, nausea, double vision, muscular weakness, and intestinal distress.

■ RDA AND DOSAGE

The RDA for vitamin E is 30 I.U. per day. Therapeutic doses in the scientific literature range from 100 I.U. to 1000 I.U. daily. Natural vitamin E (d-alpha tocopherol) is more bioavailable and, therefore, better than synthetic vitamin E (dl-alpha tocopherol).

■ FOOD SOURCES

Vitamin E is one of the most widely available nutrients in commonly available foods. Sources of vitamin E include vegetable oils, wheat germ oil, seeds, nuts, and soy beans. Other adequate sources are leafy greens, Brussels sprouts, whole-wheat products, whole-grain breads and cereals, avocados, spinach, and asparagus.

VITAMIN K

IN 1935, HENRIK DAM, a scientist in Copenhagen, Denmark, observed that newly hatched chicks receiving a diet containing all of the known essential nutrients were developing a hemorrhagic (bleeding) disease. The problem was thought to be related to a decline of prothrombin, a substance necessary for normal clotting of blood. The scientist named this newly discovered antihemmorrhagic factor vitamin K or "Koagulationsvitamin."

Vitamin K refers to a group of three vitamins called the quinones: (a) phylloquinone (K1), which occurs in green plants; (b) menaquinone (K2), which is synthesized by intestinal bacteria; and (c) menadione (K3), manufactured synthetically. The vitamin Ks are fat-soluble nutrients. Bile and pancreatic juice are necessary for their absorption from the upper small intestine, where they are carried to the liver.

■ SYMPTOMS AND CAUSES OF DEFICIENCY

Vitamin K deficiency is rare except in newborn infants. When it does occur, it can cause hemorrhaging and death. Deficiency symptoms include easy bleeding, as well as skeletal disorders such as rickets, osteoporosis, and osteomalacia.

■ BIOLOGICAL FUNCTIONS AND EFFECTS

Vitamin K is an enzymatic co-factor that is necessary for the production of a number of blood-clotting factors, including prothrombin, and factors VII, IX, and X.

Vitamin K also is necessary for the synthesis of osteocalcin, a unique protein in bone that attracts calcium to bone tissue and modulates the deposition of calcium into bone matrix. Because vitamin K plays a significant role in the calcification of bone, it may play a role in the prevention and treatment of osteoporosis.

Laboratory experiments show that vitamin K inhibits the growth of several forms of cancer, including cancers of the breast, ovary, colon, stomach, kidney, liver, and lung.

■ SIDE EFFECTS AND TOXICITY

Large doses of vitamin K can be toxic. Consequently, it is available only by prescription. In infants, vitamin K can cause a fatal form of jaundice.

■ RDA AND DOSAGE

The RDA for vitamin K is 65 mcg for women and 80 mcg for men. Pharmacologic doses in the scientific literature range from 30 to 100 mcg.

■ FOOD SOURCES

The best sources of vitamin K are liver, green leafy vegetables, and members of the cabbage family. Because intestinal bacteria synthesize vitamin K, we are not dependent upon food for this nutrient.

ZINC

Drugs that deplete zinc

■ BENAZEPRIL	■ FENOFIBRATE	■ PENICILLAMINE
■ BENZTHIAZIDE	■ FOSINOPRIL	■ POLYTHIAZIDE
■ BUMETANIDE	■ FUROSEMIDE	■ QUIONAPRIL
■ CAPTOPRIL	■ HYDROCHLORO-	■ QUINETHAZONE
■ CHLOROTHIAZIDE	THIAZIDE	■ RAMIPRIL
■ CHLORTHALIDONE	■ HYDROFLUMETHIAZIDE	■ RANITIDINE
■ CHOLESTYRAMINE	■ INDAPAMIDE	■ TETRACYCLINE
■ CIMETIDINE	■ LISINOPRIL	■ TORSEMIDE
■ CLOFIBRATE	■ METHYCLOTHIAZIDE	■ TRANDOLAPRIL
■ CORTICOSTEROIDS	■ METOLAZONE	■ TRIAMTERENE
■ ENALAPRIL	■ MOEXIPRIL	■ TRICHLOMETHIAZIDE
■ ETHACRYNIC ACID	■ NEVIRAPINE	■ VALPROIC ACID
■ ETHAMBUTOL	■ NIZATIDINE	■ ZIDOVUDINE
■ FAMOTIDINE	■ ORAL CONTRACEPTIVES	

ZINC is necessary for the functioning of well over 300 different enzymes. As such, it plays a vital role in an enormous number of biological processes. Zinc is widely distributed in microorganisms, plants, and animals. In humans, the highest concentrations of zinc are found in the liver, pancreas, kidneys, bone, and voluntary muscles. Zinc is highly concentrated in parts of the eye, prostate gland, sperm, skin, hair, and nails.

■ SYMPTOMS AND CAUSES OF DEFICIENCY

Marginal zinc deficiencies are thought to be quite common in the United States, and, because of its extensive range of biological activities, zinc deficiency can cause a wide range of deficiency symptoms. Symptoms of zinc deficiency are acne, impaired sense of smell and taste, delayed healing of wounds, anorexia, lowered immunity, frequent infections, depression, photophobia (sensitivity to light), night blindness, problems with skin, hair and nails, menstrual problems, joint pain, and nystagmus.

Zinc deficiency conditions were first reported in the 1960s in growing children and adolescent males from Egypt, Iran, and Turkey. Diets low in animal protein and high in phytate-containing grains produced symptoms of dwarfism, hypogonadism (inadequate development of sex organs), and failure to mature sexually.

Pregnant women have greater needs for zinc. Deficiency can cause impaired fetal development, infants with low birthweight, and birth defects. Stretch marks during pregnancy also are a result in part from zinc deficiency.

Zinc deficiency can be caused by inadequate dietary intake stemming from foods grown in zinc-depleted soils. Food processing also removes zinc, so fast foods and processed foods, too, are zinc-depleted. Protein- or calorie-restricted diets, too, can lead to zinc deficiency.

Zinc depletion is frequently seen in the following medical conditions:

alcoholism

macular degeneration

diabetes

malignant melanoma

liver and kidney diseases

malabsorption syndromes such as celiac sprue

inflammatory bowel diseases such as Crohn's disease.

■ BIOLOGICAL FUNCTIONS AND EFFECTS

A few of the important enzymatic activities of zinc are as follows:

- Alcohol dehydrogenase works in the liver to detoxify alcohol.
- Alkaline phosphatase frees inorganic phosphates to be used in bone metabolism.
- Carbonic anhydrase helps to excrete carbon dioxide.
- Zinc/copper-containing superoxide dismutase is a free radical scavenger.
- Cytochrome C is important in electron transport and energy production
- Carboxypeptidase is necessary for the digestion of dietary proteins.

Biological functions of zinc are as follows:

- Zinc is necessary in the synthesis of DNA and RNA, and protein, cellular division, and gene expression. Zinc protects DNA from damage.

- Zinc helps to regulate a wide variety of immune system activities, including T-lymphocytes, CD4s, natural killer cells, interleukin II, and zinc/copper superoxide dismutase.

- Zinc facilitates healing of wounds, especially in burns, surgical incisions, and other types of scars.

- Zinc enhances immune function, which makes it especially important for AIDS patients.

- Zinc gluconate lozenges reduce the length and severity of the common cold.

- Zinc is necessary for the maturation of sperm, for ovulation, and for fertilization.

- Zinc is required for normal growth and maturation.

- Zinc often is useful in treating acne and eczema.

- Zinc is a critical regulator of the sensory perceptions of taste, smell, and vision.

- Zinc controls salt-taste perception and is necessary for visual adaptation to dark and night vision.

- Zinc regulates vitamin A levels in the blood by controlling the release of stored vitamin A from the liver.

- Although zinc is a component of insulin, it does not seem to be a regulator of insulin activity.

- Zinc promotes the conversion of thyroxin to triiodothyronine.

- Because of its anti-inflammatory properties, zinc has been used successfully to treat some types of arthritis.

- Zinc is necessary for healthy prostate gland and helps to prevent benign prostatic hyperplasia (BPH).

■ SIDE EFFECTS AND TOXICITY

Zinc is relatively nontoxic, and although toxicity has been reported in humans, it is uncommon. Ingestion of high levels of zinc can induce a copper deficiency. Doses of 45 mg/day are safe, but regular intakes greater than 150 mg/day could pose a problem.

Zinc toxicity can cause diarrhea, dizziness, drowsiness, vomiting, muscular incoordination, and lethargy. Inhalation of zinc oxide in certain industrial environments also can be a source of excess exposure.

Cooking acidic foods in galvanized cookware formerly was a possible source of excess zinc intake. Widespread use of stainless steel and plastic materials to prepare and store foods has largely eliminated this problem. Galvanized pipes in older plumbing systems formerly leached zinc into drinking water supplies, but modern plumbing has phased out the use of galvanized pipes.

■ RDA AND DOSAGE

The RDA for zinc is 15 mg/day. Pharmacologic doses in the scientific literature range from 50 to 150 mg/day.

■ FOOD SOURCES

The best dietary sources of zinc are lean meats, liver, eggs, and seafood (especially oysters). Whole-grain breads and cereals are good sources of zinc.

NOTES

1. F. Nielsen et al., "Effect of Dietary Boron on Mineral, Estrogen, and Testosterone Metabolism in Postmenopausal Women," *FASEB J*, Vol. 1, No. 5 (Nov. 1987), pp. 394–397.
2. A.A. Albanese, E.J. Lorenze, H.A. Edelson et al., "Calcium Nutrition and Skeletal Bone Health," *Nutr Rep Int*, Vol. 38, No. 211, 1988.
3. R.A. Anderson and A.S. Kozlovsky, "Chromium Intake, Absorption and Excretion of Subjects Consuming Self-selected Diets," *Am J Clin Nutr*, Vol. 41, No. 6 (June 1985), pp. 1177–1183.
4. K. Lockwood, S. Moesgaard, and K. Folkers, "Partial and Complete Regression of Breast Cancer in Patients in Relation to Dosage of Coenzyme Q10," *Biochem Biophys Res Commun*, Vol. 199, No. 3 (March 30, 1994), pp. 1504–1508; S. A. Mortensen et al., "Coenzyme Q10: Clinical Benefits with Biochemical Correlates Suggesting a Scientific Breakthrough in the Management of Chronic Heart Failure," *Int J Tissue React.*, Vol. 12, No. 3 (1990), pp. 155–162.
5. W.R. Walker and D.M.Keats , "An Investigation of the Therapeutic Value of the 'Copper Bracelet'–Dermal Assimilation of Copper in Arthritic/Rheumatoid Conditions," *Agents Actions*, Vol. 6, No. 4 (July 1976), pp. 454–459.
6. J.A. Yiamouyiannis and D. Burk, "Fluoridation of Public Water Systems and the Cancer Death Rate in Humans," a paper presented at the 67th Annual Meeting of the American Society of Biologists and Chemists and the American Society of Experimental Biologists, June 1976.
7. S. Severi and G. Bedogni et al., "Effects of Home-based Food Preparation Practices on the Micronutrient Content of Foods," *European Journal of Cancer Prevention*, Vol. 7, No. 4, 1998, pp. 331–335.
8. E.M. Pao and S.J. Mickle, "Problem Nutrients in the United States," *Food Technology*, Vol. 35, 1981, pp. 58–62.
9. Z.Y. Zhao, Y. Xie et al., "Aging and the Circadian Rhythm of Melatonin: A Cross-sectional Study of Chinese Subjects 30–110 Yr of Age," *Chronobiol Int.*, Vol, 19. No. 6 (Nov. 2002), pp. 1171–1182.

10. K.T. Khaw and E. Barrett–Connor, "Dietary Potassium and Stroke-associated Mortality. A 12-year Prospective Population Study," *New England Journal of Medicine*, Vol. 316, No. 5, (Jan. 29, 1987), pp. 235–240.
11. M. Poa and S.J. Mickle, "Problem Nutrients in the United States," *Food Technology,* Vol. 35, 1981, pp. 58–62.
12. P.L. Canner, K.G. Berge, and N.K. Wenger et al., "Fifteen Year Mortality in Coronary Drug Project Patients: Long-term Benefit with Niacin," *J Am Coll Cardiol.*, Vol. 8, 1986, pp. 1245–1255.
13. Linus Pauling, *How To Live Longer and Feel Better.* New York: W.H. Freeman and Company, 1986, p. 120.
14. H.M. Evans and H. M., Bishop, "Fetal Resorption," *Science,* Vol. 55, 1922, p. 650.

This Part provides a guide to brand names and the corresponding generic names of drugs. The first column gives the registered or trademarked name of the drug. The second column designates the corresponding generic name or category of drug discussed in this book. Readers may find that a drug they are taking is not mentioned here. This means that no studies have been conducted to evaluate whether the drug causes nutrient depletion — which is particularly true of many of the newer drugs on the market. OTC designates over-the counter drugs. Those not so designated are prescription drugs.

BRAND NAMES/
GENERIC NAMES

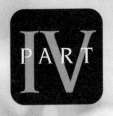

PART

IV

Abelcet® Injection / *Amphotericin B*
Accupril® / *Quinapril*
Aceon® / *Perindopril erbumine*
Aches-N-Pain® (OTC) / *NSAIDs*
Achromycin® Ophthalmic / *Tetracyclines*
Achromycin® Topical / *Tetracyclines*
Aciphex® / *Rabeprazole*
Acticort 100® / *Corticosteroids*
Actron® (OTC) / *NSAIDs*
Acular® Ophthalmic / *NSAIDs*
Adalat® / *Nifedipine*
Adalat® CC / *Nifedipine*
Adapin® Oral / *Doxepin*
Adlone® Injection / *Corticosteroids*
Adprin-B®, Extra Strength (OTC) / *Aspirin*
Adriamycin PFS™ / *Chemotherapy drug*
Adriamycin RFD® / *Chemotherapy drug*
Adrucil® Injection / *Chemotherapy drug*
Advil® (OTC) / *NSAIDs*
Advil®, Children's, Oral Suspension / *NSAIDs*
AeroBid-M® Oral Aerosol Inhaler /
   Corticosteroids
AeroBid® Oral Aerosol Inhaler /
   Corticosteroids
Aerolate III® / *Theophylline*
Aerolate Jr® / *Theophylline*
Aerolate Sr® / *Theophylline*
Aeroseb-Dex® / *Corticosteroids*
Aeroseb-HC® / *Corticosteroids*
Agoral Plain® (OTC) / *Mineral oil*
A-hydroCort® / *Corticosteroids*
Airet® / *Albuterol*
AK-Dex® / *Corticosteroids*
AK-Pred® Ophthalmic / *Corticosteroids*
AKTob® Ophthalmic / *Aminoglycosides*
Ala-Cort® / *Corticosteroids*
Ala-Scalp® / *Corticosteroids*
Alba-Dex® / *Corticosteroids*
Aldomet® / *Methyldopa*
Alesse™ / *Oral contraceptives*
Aleve® (OTC) / *NSAIDs*
Alkaban-AQ® / *Chemotherapy drug*
Alkaren® / *Chemotherapy drug*
Alphatrex® / *Corticosteroids*
Altace® / *Ramipril*
ALternaGEL® (OTC) / *Aluminum hydroxide*
Alu-Cap® (OTC) / *Aluminum hydroxide*
Aludrox® (OTC) / *Aluminum hydroxide and
   magnesium hydroxide*
Alu-Tab® (OTC) / *Aluminum hydroxide*
AmBisome® / *Amphotericin B*
Amcort® / *Corticosteroids*
A-methaPred® Injection / *Corticosteroids*

Amikin® Injection / *Aminoglycosides*
Amoxil® / *Penicillins*
Amphocin® / *Amphotericin B*
Amphojel® (OTC) / *Aluminum hydroxide*
Amytal® / *Barbiturates*
Anacin® (OTC) / *Aspirin*
Anafranil® / *Clomipramine*
Anaprox® / *NSAIDs*
Ancef® / *Cephalosporin*
Anergan® / *Promethazine*
Anucort-HC® Suppository / *Corticosteroids*
Anuprep HC® Suppository / *Corticosteroids*
Anusol® HC-1 (OTC) / *Corticosteroids*
Anusol® HC-2.5% (OTC) / *Corticosteroids*
Anusol-HC® Suppository / *Corticosteroids*
Apresazide® / *Hydralazine and
   hydrochlorothiazide*
Apresoline® / *Hydralazine*
Aquaphyllin® / *Theophylline*
Aquatag® / *Benzthiazide*
Aquatensen® / *Methyclothiazide*
Argesic®-SA / *Salsalate*
Aristocort® / *Corticosteroids*
Aristocort® A / *Corticosteroids*
Aristocort Forte® / *Corticosteroids*
Aristocort® Intralesional / *Corticosteroids*
Aristospan® Intra-Articular / *Corticosteroids*
Aristospan® Intralesional / *Corticosteroids*
Artha-G® / *Salsalate*
Arthritis Foundation® Pain Reliever (OTC) /
   Aspirin
Arthropan® (OTC) / *Choline salicylate*
Articulose-50® Injection / *Corticosteroids*
Ascriptin® (OTC) / *Aspirin*
Asendin® / *Amoxapine*
Asmalix® / *Theophylline*
Aspergum® (OTC) / *Salicylates*
Asprimox® (OTC) / *Aspirin*
Atarax® / *Hydroxyzine*
Atolone® / *Corticosteroids*
Atridox® / *Doxycycline*
Atromid-S® / *Clofibrate*
Augmentin® / *Penicillins*
Aureomycin® / *Chlortetracycline*
Aventyl® / *Hydrochloride nortriptyline*
Axid® / *Nizatidine*
Axid® AR (OTC) / *Nizatidine*
Azmacort™ / *Corticosteroids*
Azulfidine® / *Sulfasalazine*
Azulfidine® EN tabs / *Sulfasalazine*

Bactocill® / *Penicillins*
Bactrim™ / *Co-Trimoxazole*

Bactrim™ DS / *Co-Trimoxazole*
Baldex® / *Corticosteroids*
Barbita® / *Barbiturates*
Baycol® / *Cerivastatin*
Bayer®Aspirin (OTC) / *Aspirin*
Bayer® Buffered Aspirin (OTC) / *Aspirin*
Bayer® Enteric 500 Aspirin, Extra
   Strength (OTC) / *Aspirin*
Bayer® Enteric 500 Aspirin, Regular
   Strength (OTC) / *Aspirin*
Bayer ® Low Adult Strength (OTC) / *Aspirin*
Bayer® Plus, Extra Strength (OTC) / *Aspirin*
Beepen-VK® / *Penicillins*
Betapace® / *Beta-blockers*
Betapen®-VK / *Penicillins*
Betatrex® / *Corticosteroids*
Beta-Val® / *Corticosteroids*
Betimol® Ophthalmic / *Beta-blockers*
Betoptic® Ophthalmic / *Beta-blockers*
Biaxin® / *Macrolide*
Bicillin® C-R / *Penicillins*
Bicillin® C-R 900/300 / *Penicillins*
Bicillin® L-A / *Penicillins*
BiCNU® / *Chemotherapy drug*
Biomox® / *Penicillins*
Bio-Tab® / *Doxycycline*
Bisac-Evac® (OTC) / *Bisacodyl*
Bisacodyl Uniserts® / *Bisacodyl*
Bisco-Lax® / *Bisacodyl*
Blocadren® Oral / *Beta-blockers*
Brethaire® Inhalation Aerosol / *Terbutaline*
Brethine® Injection / *Terbutaline*
Brethine® Oral / *Terbutaline*
Brevibloc® Injection / *Beta-blockers*
Brevicon® / *Oral contraceptives*
Brevital® / *Barbiturates*
Bricanyl® Injection / *Terbutaline*
Bricanyl® Oral / *Terbutaline*
Bronkodyl® / *Theophylline*
Bufferin® (OTC) / *Aspirin*
Buffex® (OTC) / *Aspirin*
Bumex® / *Bumetanide*
Butalan® / *Barbiturates*
Buticaps® / *Barbiturates*
Butisol Sodium® / *Barbiturates*

Calan® / *Verapamil*
Calan® SR / *Verapamil*
CaldeCORT® / *Corticosteroids*
CaldeCORT® Anti-Itch Spray / *Corticosteroids*
Cama® Arthritis Pain Reliever / *Aspirin*
Camptosar® / *Chemotherapy drugs*
Capoten® / *Captopril*

Carbatrol® / *Carbamazepine*
Cardene® / *Calcium channel blockers*
Cardizem® / *Calcium channel blockers*
Carter's Little Pills® (OTC) / *Bisacodyl*
Cartrol® Oral / *Beta-blockers*
Cataflam® Oral / *NSAIDs*
Catapres® Oral / *Clonidine*
Catapres-TTS® Transdermal / *Clonidine*
Ceclor® / *Cephalosporin*
Ceclor® CD / *Cephalosporins*
Cedax® / *Cephalosporins*
CeeNU® / *Chemotherapy drug*
Cefobid® / *Cephalosporins*
Cefotan® / *Cephalosporins*
Ceftin® Oral / *Cephalosporins*
Cefzil® / *Cephalosporins*
Celebrex™ / *Celecoxib*
Celestone® / *Corticosteroids*
Celestone® Soluspan / *Corticosteroids*
Celexa® / *Citalopram*
Celontin® / *Methsuximide*
Cel-U-Jec® / *Corticosteroids*
Cena-K® (TR) / *Potassium chloride*
Ceptaz™ / *Cephalosporins*
Cerebyx® / *Fosphenytoin*
Cetacort® / *Corticosteroids*
Chibroxin™ Ophthalmic / *Fluoroquinolone*
Ciloxan™ Ophthalmic / *Fluoroquinolone*
Cipro™ / *Fluoroquinolone*
Cipro™ IV / *Fluoroquinolone*
Claforan® / *Cephalosporins*
Clinoril® / *NSAIDs*
Clocort®Maximum Strength / *Corticosteroids*
Clysodrast® / *Bisacodyl*
Col-benemid® / *Colchicine*
Colestid® / *Colestipol*
CombiPatch® / *Oral contraceptives*
Compazine® / *Prochlorperazine*
Coreg® / *Beta-blockers*
Corgard® / *Beta-blockers*
CortaGel® (OTC) / *Corticosteroids*
Cortaid® Maximum Strength (OTC) /
   Corticosteroids
Cortaid® With Aloe / *Corticosteroids*
Cort-Dome® / *Corticosteroids*
Cortef® / *Corticosteroids*
Cortef® Feminine Itch / *Corticosteroids*
Cortenema® / *Corticosteroids*
Cortifoam® / *Corticosteroids*
Cortizone®-5 (OTC) / *Corticosteroids*
Cortizone®-10 (OTC) / *Corticosteroids*
Cortone®Acetate / *Corticosteroids*
Cosmegen® / *Chemotherapy drug*

Cotrim® / *Co-Trimoxazole*
Cotrim® DS / *Co-Trimoxazole*
Covera-HS® / *Verapamil*
Crestor® / *Rosuvastatin calcium*
Crysticillin® AS / *Penicillins*
Cuprimine® / *Penicillamine*
Cutivate™ / *Corticosteroids*
Cytosar-U® / *Chemotherapy drug*
Cytoxan® Oral / *Chemotherapy drug*
Cytoxan® Injection / *Chemotherapy drug*

Dacodyl® (OTC) / *Bisacodyl*
Dalalone L.A.® / *Corticosteroids*
DaunoXome® / *Chemotherapy drug*
Decaderm® / *Corticosteroids*
Decadron® / *Corticosteroids*
Decadron® LA / *Corticosteroids*
Decadron® Turbinaire / *Corticosteroids*
Decaject-L.A.® / *Corticosteroids*
Decaspray® / *Corticosteroids*
Declomycin® / *Demeclocycline*
Deficol® / *Bisacodyl*
Dekasol-L.A.® / *Corticosteroids*
Delcort® / *Corticosteroids*
Delta-Cortef® Oral / *Corticosteroids*
Deltasone® / *Corticosteroids*
Delta-Tritex® / *Corticosteroids*
Demadex® / *Torsemide*
Demulen® / *Oral contraceptives*
Depacon® / *Valproic acid*
Depakene® / *Valproic acid*
Depakote® / *Valproic acid*
Depen® / *Penicillamine*
DepMedalone® / *Corticosteroids*
Depoject® Injection / *Corticosteroids*
Depo-Medrol® Injection / *Corticosteroids*
Depopred® Injection / *Corticosteroids*
Dermacort® / *Corticosteroids*
Dermarest Dricort® / *Corticosteroids*
DermiCort® / *Corticosteroids*
Dermolate® (OTC) / *Corticosteroids*
Dermtex® / *Corticosteroids*
Desogen® / *Oral contraceptives*
Dexair® / *Corticosteroids*
Dexasone LA® / *Corticosteroids*
Dexone® / *Corticosteroids*
Dexone LA® / *Corticosteroids*
Dezone® / *Corticosteroids*
Diabeta® / *Glyburide*
Dialume® / *Aluminum hydroxide*
Di-Gel® (OTC) / *Aluminum hydroxide, magnesium hydroxide, and simethicone*
Dilacor® / *Calcium channel blockers*

Dilantin® / *Phenytoin*
Diphenylan Sodium® / *Phenytoin*
Diprolene® / *Corticosteroids*
Diprolene® AF / *Corticosteroids*
Diprosone® / *Corticosteroids*
Disalcid® / *Salsalate*
Diucardin® / *Hydroflumethiazide*
Diurigen® / *Chlorothiazide*
Diuril® / *Chlorothiazide*
D-Med® Injection / *Corticosteroids*
Dolobid® / *NSAIDs*
Dopar® / *Levodopa*
Doryx® / *Doxycycline*
Doxy® / *Doxycycline*
Doxychel® / *Doxycycline*
Droxia™ / *Chemotherapy drug*
DTIC-Dome® / *Chemotherapy drug*
Dulcolax® (OTC) / *Bisacodyl*
Duraclon® / *Clonidine*
Duralone® Injection / *Corticosteroids*
Duricef® / *Cephalosporin*
Dyazide® / *Hydrochlorothiazide and Triamterene*
Dycill® / *Penicillins*
Dymelor® / *Acetohexamide*
Dynabac® / *Macrolides*
Dynacin® Oral / *Minocycline*
Dynapen® / *Penicillins*
Dyrenium® / *Triamterene*

Easprin® / *Aspirin*
E-Base® / *Macrolides*
Econopred® Ophthalmic / *Corticosteroids*
Econopred® Plus Ophthalmic / *Corticosteroids*
Ecotrin® (OTC) / *Aspirin*
Ecotrin® Low Adult Strength (OTC) / *Aspirin*
Edecrin® / *Ethacrynic acid*
E.E.S.® / *Macrolides*
Efudex® Topical / *Chemotherapy drug*
Elavil® / *Amitriptyline*
Eldecort® / *Corticosteroids*
Elixomin® / *Theophylline*
Elixophyllin® / *Theophylline*
Elocon® Topical / *Corticosteroids*
Elspar® / *Chemotherapy drug*
Eltroxin® / *Levothyroxine*
Empirin® (OTC) / *Aspirin*
E-Mycin® / *Macrolides*
Enduron® / *Methyclothiazide*
Enovil® / *Amitriptyline*
Epitol® / *Carbamazepine*
Epivir® / *Lamivudine*
Epivir® HBV / *Lamivudine*

Eramycin® / *Macrolides*
Eryc® / *Macrolides*
EryPed® / *Macrolides*
Ery-Tab® / *Macrolides*
Erythrocin® / *Macrolides*
Esidrix® / *Hydrochlorothiazide*
Eskalith® / *Lithium*
Eskalith® CR / *Lithium*
Estratab® / *Estrogens, esterified*
Estrostep® / *Oral contraceptives*
Estrostep® Fe / *Oral contraceptives*
Excedrin® IB (OTC) / *NSAIDs*
Exna® / *Benzthiazide*
Ezide® / *Hydrochlorothiazide*

Feen-A-Mint® / *Bisacodyl*
Feldene® / *NSAIDs*
Fleet® Laxative (OTC) / *Bisacodyl*
Fleet®Mineral Oil Enema (OTC) / *Mineral oil*
Flonase® / *Corticosteroids*
Fluoroplex® Topical / *Chemotherapy drug*
Flovent® / *Corticosteroids*
Floxin® / *Fluoroquinolones*
Fludara® / *Chemotherapy drug*
Flutex® / *Corticosteroids*
Folex® / *Methotrexate*
Fortaz® / *Cephalosporins*
Foscavir® Injection / *Foscarnet*
FUDR® / *Chemotherapy drug*
Fungizone® / *Amphotericin B*

Gantanol® / *Sulfonamides*
Garamycin® / *Aminoglycosides*
Gas-Ban DS® (OTC) / *Aluminum hydroxide, magnesium hydroxide, and simethicone*
Gaviscon®-2 Tablet (OTC) / *Aluminum hydroxide and magnesium trisilicate*
Gaviscon® Liquid (OTC) / *Aluminum hydroxide and magnesium carbonate*
Gaviscon® Tablet (OTC) / *Aluminum hydroxide and magnesium trisilicate*
Gelusil® (OTC) / *Aluminum hydroxide, magnesium hydroxide, and simethicone*
Gemcor® / *Gemfibrozil*
Gemzar® / *Chemotherapy drug*
Gen-K® (TR) / *Potassium chloride*
Genoptic® Ophthalmic / *Aminoglycosides*
Genoptic®SOP Ophthalmic / *Aminoglycosides*
Genora® / *Oral contraceptives*
Genora® 1/35 / *Oral contraceptives*
Genora® 1/50 / *Oral contraceptives*
Genpril® (OTC) / *NSAIDs*
Gentacidin® Ophthalmic / *Aminoglycosides*

Gentafair® / *Aminoglycosides*
Gentak® Ophthalmic / *Aminoglycosides*
Gentrasul® / *Aminoglycosides*
Geocillin® / *Penicillins*
Glucophage® / *Metformin*
Glynase™ PresTab® / *Glyburide*
G-myticin® Topical / *Aminoglycosides*
Gynecort® (OTC) / *Corticosteroids*

Haldol® / *Haloperidol*
Haldol® Decanoate / *Haloperidol*
Haley's M-O® / *Mineral oil*
Halfprin® 81 (OTC) / *Aspirin*
Haltran® (OTC) / *NSAIDs*
Hemril-HC® Uniserts® / *Corticosteroids*
Hexadrol® / *Corticosteroids*
Hi-Cor-1.0® / *Corticosteroids*
Hi-Cor-2.5® / *Corticosteroids*
Hivid® / *Zalcitabine*
Hycamtin™ / *Chemotherapy drug*
Hycort® / *Corticosteroids*
Hydrap-ES® / *Hydralazine, hydrochlorothiazide, and reserpine*
Hydrea® / *Chemotherapy drug*
Hydrex® / *Benzthiazide*
Hydrocort® / *Corticosteroids*
Hydrocortone® Acetate / *Corticosteroids*
Hydrocortone® Phosphate / *Corticosteroids*
HydroDIURIL® / *Hydrochlorothiazide*
Hydromox® / *Quinethazone*
Hydro-Par® / *Hydrochlorothiazide*
HydroSKIN® / *Corticosteroids*
Hydro-Tex® (OTC) / *Corticosteroids*
Hygroton® / *Chlorthalidone*
Hytone® / *Corticosteroids*

Ibuprin® (OTC) / *NSAIDs*
Ibuprohm® / *NSAIDs*
Ibu-Tab® / *NSAIDs*
Idamycin® / *Chemotherapy drug*
Ifex® / *Chemotherapy drug*
I-Gent® / *Aminoglycosides*
Ilosone® / *Macrolides*
I-Methasone® / *Corticosteroids*
Inderal® / *Proprandolol*
Indochron E-R® / *NSAIDs*
Indocin® / *NSAIDs*
Indocin® IV / *Indomethacin*
Indocin® SR / *NSAIDs*
Inflamase® Forte Ophthalmic / *Corticosteroids*
Inflamase® Mild Ophthalmic / *Corticosteroids*
Isoptin® / *Verapamil*
Isoptin® SR / *Verapamil*

Janimine® / *Imipramine*
Jenamicin® Injection / *Aminoglycosides*
Jenest-28™ / *Oral contraceptives*

K+ 10® (TR) / *Potassium chloride*
Kantrex® / *Aminoglycosides*
Kaochlor® (TR) / *Potassium chloride*
Kaochlor® SF (TR) / *Potassium chloride*
Kaon-Cl® (TR) / *Potassium chloride*
Kaon Cl-10® (TR) / *Potassium chloride*
Kay Ciel® (TR) / *Potassium chloride*
K+ Care® (TR) / *Potassium chloride*
K-Dur® 10 (TR) / *Potassium chloride*
K-Dur® 20 (TR) / *Potassium chloride*
Keflex® / *Cephalosporins*
Keftab® / *Cephalosporins*
Kefurox® Injection / *Cephalosporins*
Kefzol® / *Cephalosporins*
Kenacort® / *Corticosteroids*
Kenaject-40® / *Corticosteroids*
Kenalog® / *Corticosteroids*
Kenalog-10® / *Corticosteroids*
Kenalog-40® / *Corticosteroids*
Kenalog® H / *Corticosteroids*
Kenalog® in Orabase® / *Corticosteroids*
Kenonel® / *Corticosteroids*
Kerlone® Oral / *Beta-blockers*
Key-Pred® Injection / *Corticosteroids*
Key-Pred-SP® Injection / *Corticosteroids*
K-Lease® (TR) / *Potassium chloride*
K-Lor® (TR) / *Potassium chloride*
Klor-Con® (TR) / *Potassium chloride*
Klor-Con® 8 (TR) / *Potassium chloride*
Klor-Con® 10 (TR) / *Potassium chloride*
Klor-Con/25® / *Potassium chloride*
Klorvess® (TR) / *Potassium chloride*
Klotrix® (TR) / *Potassium chloride*
K-Lyte/Cl® (TR) / *Potassium chloride*
K-Norm® (TR) / *Potassium chloride*
Kondremul® (OTC) / *Mineral oil*
K-Tab® (TR) / *Potassium chloride*

LactiCare-HC® / *Corticosteroids*
Lanacort® (OTC) / *Corticosteroids*
Laniazid® Oral / *Isoniazid*
Lanophyllin® / *Theophylline*
Lanoxicaps® / *Digoxin*
Lanoxin® / *Digoxin*
Larodopa® / *Levodopa*
Lasix® / *Furosemide*
L-Dopa® / *Levodopa*
Lescol® / *Fluvastatin*
Leustatin® / *Chemotherapy drug*

Levaquin™ / *Fluoroquinolone*
Levlen® / *Oral contraceptives*
Levoprome® / *Methotrimeprazine*
Levora® / *Oral contraceptives*
Levo-T™ / *Levothyroxine*
Levothroid® / *Levothyroxine*
Levoxyl® / *Levothyroxine*
Lipitor® / *Atorvastatin*
Liquid Pred® / *Corticosteroids*
Lithane® / *Lithium*
Lithobid® / *Lithium*
Lithonate® / *Lithium*
Lithotabs® / *Lithium*
Locoid® / *Corticosteroids*
Lodine® / *NSAIDs*
Lodine® XL / *NSAIDs*
Loestrin® / *Oral contraceptives*
Loestrin® Fe / *Oral contraceptives*
Lo/Ovral® / *Oral contraceptives*
Lopid® / *Gemfibrozil*
Lopressor® / *Beta-blockers*
Lorabid® / *Cephalosporins*
Lotensin® / *Benazepril*
Lozol® / *Indapamide*
Lukeran® / *Chemotherapy drug*
Luminal® / *Barbiturates*
Luvox® / *Fluvoxamine*
Lysodren® / *Chemotherapy drug*

Maalox® (OTC) / *Aluminum hydroxide and magnesium* hydroxide
Maalox® Plus (OTC) / *Aluminum hydroxide, magnesium hydroxide, and simethicone*
Maalox® Therapeutic Concentrate (OTC) / *Aluminum hydroxide and magnesium hydroxide*
Magalox Plus® (OTC) / *Aluminum hydroxide, magnesium hydroxide, and simethicone*
Mandol® / *Cephalosporin*
Maox® / *Magnesium oxide*
Marazide® / *Benzthiazide*
Marcillin® / *Penicillin*
Marpres® / *Hydralazine, hydrochlorothiazide, and reserpine*
Marthritic® / *Salsalate*
Mavik® / *Trandolapril*
Maxaquin® / *Fluoroquinolones*
Maxidex® / *Corticosteroids*
Maxipime® / *Cephalosporins*
Maxivate® / *Corticosteroid*
Maxzide® / *Hydrochlorothiazide and triamterene*
Mebaral® / *Barbiturates*

Meclomen® / *NSAIDs*
Medipren® / *NSAIDs*
Medralone® / *Corticosteroids*
Medrol® / *Corticosteroids*
Mefoxin® / *Cephalosporins*
Mellaril® / *Thioridazine*
Mellaril-S® / *Thioridazine*
Menadol® (OTC) / *NSAIDs*
Menest® / *Estrogen, esterified*
Metahydrin® / *Trichlormethiazide*
Methylone® / *Corticosteroids*
Meticorten® / *Corticosteroids*
Metreton® Ophthalmic / *Corticosteroids*
Mevacor® / *Lovastatin*
Mezlin® / *Penicillins*
Micro-K® 10 (TR) / *Potassium chloride*
Micro-K® Extencaps® (TR) / *Potassium chloride*
Micro-K® LS® (TR) / *Potassium chloride*
Micronase® / *Glyburide*
Microsulfon® / *Sulfonamides*
Microzide™ / *Hydrochlorothiazide*
Midamor® / *Amiloride*
Midol® 200 (OTC) / *NSAIDs*
Milkinol® (OTC) / *Mineral oil*
Minocin® IV Injection / *Minocycline*
Minocin® Oral / *Minocycline*
Mircette™ / *Oral contraceptives*
Mithracin® / *Chemotherapy drug*
Modicon™ / *Oral contraceptives*
Mono-Gesic® / *Salsalate*
Monopril® / *Fosinopril*
Motrin® / *NSAIDs*
Motrin®, Children's, Oral Suspension / *NSAIDs*
Motrin® IB (OTC) / *NSAIDs*
Motrin®, Junior Strength (OTC) / *NSAIDs*
M-Prednisol® Injection / *Corticosteroids*
Mustargen® / *Hydrochloride*
Mutamycin® / *Chemotherapy drug*
Myambutol® / *Ethambutol*
Mycifradin® Sulfate Oral / *Neomycin*
Mycifradin® Sulfate / *Neomycin, topical*
Mylanta® (OTC) / *Aluminum hydroxide, magnesium hydroxide, and simethicone*
Mylanta®-II (OTC) / *Aluminum hydroxide, magnesium hydroxide, and simethicone*
Myleran® / *Chemotherapy drug*
Mysoline® / *Primidone*

Nafcil™ Injection / *Penicillin*
Nalfon® / *NSAIDs*
Nallpen® Injection / *Penicillins*
Naprelan® / *NSAIDs*

Naprosyn® / *NSAIDs*
Naqua® / *Trichlormethiazide*
Nardil® / *Phelelzine*
Nasacort® / *Corticosteroids*
Nasacort® AQ / *Corticosteroids*
Nasalide® Nasal Aerosol / *Corticosteroids*
Nasarel™ / *Corticosteroids*
Navelbine® / *Chemotherapy drug*
Nebcin® Injection / *Aminoglycoside*
NebuPent® Inhalation / *Pentamidine*
N.E.E.® 1/35 / *Oral contraceptives*
Nelova™ 0.5/35E / *Oral contraceptives*
Nelova™ 1/35E / *Oral contraceptives*
Nelova™ 1/50M / *Oral contraceptives*
Nelova™ 10/11 / *Oral contraceptives*
Nembutal® / *Barbiturates*
Neo-Cultol® (OTC) / *Mineral oil*
Neo-fradin® Oral / *Neomycin*
Neo-Tabs® Oral / *Neomycin*
Neut® Injection / *Sodium bicarbonate*
Nexium® / *Esomeprazole*
Nordette® / *Oral contraceptives*
Norethin™ 1/35E / *Oral contraceptives*
Norethin™ 1/50M / *Oral contraceptives*
Norinyl® 1+35, / *Oral contraceptives*
Norinyl® 1+50 / *Oral contraceptives*
Normodyne® / *Beta-blockers*
Noroxin® Oral / *Fluoroquinolone*
Norpramin® / *Desipramine*
Nor-tet® Oral / *Tetracycline*
Norvasc® / *Calcium channel blockers*
Norzine® / *Thiethylperazine*
Nuprin® (OTC) / *NSAIDs*
Nutracort® / *Corticosteroids*
Novantrone® / *Chemotherapy drug*
Nydrazid® Injection / *Isoniazid*

Ocu-Dex® / *Corticosteroids*
Ocuflox™ Ophthalmic / *Fluoroquinolones*
Ocumycin® / *Aminoglycosides*
Ocupress® / *Beta-blockers*
Omnipen® / *Penicillins*
Omnipen®-N / *Penicillins*
Oncovin® Injection / *Chemotherapy drug*
Orabase® HCA / *Corticosteroids*
Orasone® / *Corticosteroids*
Oretic® / *Hydrochlorothiazide*
Ortho® 0.5/35 / *Oral contraceptives*
Ortho-Cept® / *Oral contraceptives*
Ortho-Cyclen® / *Oral contraceptives*
Ortho-Novum® 1/35 / *Oral contraceptives*
Ortho-Novum® 1/50 / *Oral contraceptives*
Ortho-Novum® 7/7/7 / *Oral contraceptives*

Ortho-Novum® 10/11 / *Oral contraceptives*
Ortho Tri-Cyclen® / *Oral contraceptives*
Orudis® / *NSAIDs*
Orudis® KT (OTC) / *NSAIDs*
Oruvail® / *NSAIDs*
Ovcon® 35 / *Oral contraceptives*
Ovcon® 50 / *Oral contraceptives*
Ovral® / *Oral contraceptives*
Ovrette® / *Oral contraceptive*

Pamelor® / *Nortriptyline*
Pamprin IB® (OTC) / *NSAIDs*
Pandel® / *Corticosteroids*
Panmycin® Oral / *Tetracyclines*
Paraplatin® / *Chemotherapy drug*
Pathocil® / *Penicillins*
Paxene® / *Chemotherapy drugs*
Paxil® / *Paroxetine*
PCE® / *Macrolides*
Pediapred® Oral / *Corticosteroids*
PediaProfen™ / *NSAIDs*
Penecort® / *Corticosteroids*
Pentacarinat® / *Pentamidine*
Pentam-300® Injection / *Pentamidine*
Pentothal® / *Barbiturates*
Pen.Vee K® / *Penicillins*
Pepcid® / *Famotidine*
Pepcid® AC Acid Controller / *Famotidine*
Periostat™ / *Doxycycline*
Permapen® / *Penicillins*
Permitil®Oral / *Fluphenazine*
Pfizerpen® / *Penicillin*
Phenazine® / *Promethazine*
Phenergan® / *Promethazine*
Phillips'® Milk of Magnesia (OTC) /
   Magnesium hydroxide
Pipracil® / *Penicillins*
Plaquenil® / *Hydroxychloroquine*
Platinol® / *Chemotherapy drug*
Platinol®-AQ / *Chemotherapy drug*
Plendil® / *Calcium channel blockers*
Polycillin® / *Penicillins*
Polycillin-N® / *Penicillins*
Polymox® / *Penicillins*
Ponstel® / *NSAIDs*
Potasalan®(TR) / *Potassium chloride*
Pravachol® / *Pravastatin*
Predair® / *Corticosteroids*
Predaject® / *Corticosteroids*
Predalone TBA® / *Corticosteroids*
Predcor® / *Corticosteroids*
Predcor-TBA® / *Corticosteroids*
Pred Forte® Ophthalmic / *Corticosteroids*

Pred Mild® Ophthalmic / *Corticosteroids*
Prednicen-M® / *Corticosteroids*
Prednisol® TBA Injection / *Corticosteroids*
Prelone® Oral / *Corticosteroids*
Premarin® / *Estrogens, conjugated*
Premphase™ / *Estrogen and
   medroxyprogesterone*
Prempro™ / *Estrogen and medroxyprogesterone*
Pre-Par® / *Ritodrine*
Prevacid® / *Lansoprazole*
Prevalite® / *Cholestyramine resin*
Prilosec™ / *Omeprazole*
Principen® / *Penicillins*
Prinivil® / *Lisinopril*
Proaqua® / *Benzthiazide*
Procardia® / *Nifedipine*
Procardia® XL / *Nifedipine*
Procort® (OTC) / *Corticosteroids*
Proctocort™ / *Corticosteroids*
Prolixin Decanoate® Injection / *Fluphenazine*
Prolixin Enanthate® Injection / *Fluphenazine*
Prolixin® Injection / *Fluphenazine*
Prolixin® Oral / *Fluphenazine*
Proloprim® / *Trimethoprim*
Prorex® / *Promethazine*
Prostaphlin® / *Penicillins*
Protonix® / *Pantoprazole*
Proventil® / *Albuterol*
Prozac® / *Fluoxetine*
Psorion® Cream / *Corticosteroids*
Pulmicort Turbuhaler® / *Corticosteroids*
Purinethol® / *Chemotherapy drug*

Questran® / *Cholestyramine resin*
Questran® Light / *Cholestyramine resin*
Quibron®-T / *Theophylline*
Quibron®-T/SR / *Theophylline*

Raxar® / *Fluoroquinolone*
Relafen® / *NSAIDs*
Renese® / *Polythiazide*
Rescriptor® / *Delavirdine*
Respbid® / *Theophylline*
Retrovir® / *Zidovudine*
Rheumatrex® / *Methotrexate*
Rhinocort® / *Corticosteroids*
Rifadin® / *Rifampin*
Rifadin® Injection / *Rifampin*
Rifadin® Oral / *Rifampin*
Rimactane® / *Rifampin*
Rimactane® Oral / *Rifampin*
Robicillin® VK / *Penicillins*
Rocephin® / *Cephalosporin*

Rubex® / *Chemotherapy drug*
Rum-K® / *Potassium chloride TR*

Saleto-200® (OTC) / *NSAIDs*
Saleto-400® / *NSAIDs*
Salflex® / *Salsalate*
Salgesic® / *Salsalate*
Salsitab® / *Salsalate*
Saluron® / *Hydroflumethiazide*
Scalpicin® / *Corticosteroids*
Seconal™ / *Barbiturates*
Sectral® / *Beta-blockers*
Septra® / *Sulfonamides*
Septra® DS / *Sulfonamides*
Ser-Ap-Es® / *Hydralazine, hydrochlorothiazide,
    and reserpine*
Serentil® / *Mesoridazine*
Sertan® / *Primidone*
Seromycin® / *Antibiotics*
Sinequan® Oral / *Doxepin*
Slo-bid™ / *Theophylline*
Slo-Phyllin® / *Theophylline*
Slow-K® / *Potassium chloride* **TR**
Solfoton® / *Barbiturates*
Solu-Cortef® / *Corticosteroids*
Solu-Medrol® Injection / *Corticosteroids*
Solurex L.A.® / *Corticosteroids*
Sotalol® / *Beta-blockers*
Sparine® / *Promazine*
Spectrobid® / *Penicillins*
S-T Cort® / *Corticosteroids*
Stelazine® / *Trifluoperazine*
Sterapred® / *Corticosteroids*
Stilphostrol® / *Diethylstilbestrol*
St Joseph® Adult Chewable Aspirin (OTC) /
    Aspirin
Sulfatrim® / *Co-trimoxazole*
Sumycin® Oral / *Tetracyclines*
Suprax® / *Cephalosporins*
Surmontil® / *Trimipramine*
Sustaire® / *Theophylline*
Synacort® / *Corticosteroids*
Synthroid® / *Levothyroxine*

Tac™-3 / *Corticosteroids*
Tac™-40 / *Corticosteroids*
Tacaryl® / *Methdilazine*
TACE® / *Chlorotrianisene*
Tagamet® / *Cimetidine*
Tagamet® HB (OTC) / *Cimetidine*
Taxol® / *Chemotherapy drug*
Taxotere® / *Chemotherapy drug*
Tazicef® / *Cephalosporins*

Tazidime® / *Cephalosporins*
Tegretol® / *Carbamazepine*
Tegretol®-XR / *Carbamazepine*
Tegrin®-HC (OTC) / *Corticosteroids*
Teladar® / *Corticosteroids*
Ten-K® / *Potassium chloride* **TR**
Tenormin® / *Beta-blockers*
Terramycin® I.M. Injection / *Oxytetracycline*
Terramycin® Oral / *Oxytetracycline*
Tetracap® Oral / *Tetracyclines*
Thalitone® / *Chlorthalidone*
Theo-24® / *Theophylline*
Theobid® / *Theophylline*
Theochron® / *Theophylline*
Theoclear-80® / *Theophylline*
Theoclear L.A.® / *Theophylline*
Theo-Dur® / *Theophylline*
Theolair™ / *Theophylline*
Theo-Sav® / *Theophylline*
Theospan-SR® / *Theophylline*
Theostat-80® / *Theophylline*
Theovent® / *Theophylline*
Theo-X® / *Theophylline*
Thorazine® / *Chlorpromazine*
Tiazac® / *Calcium channel blockers*
Ticar® / *Penicillins*
Timoptic® OcuDose® / *Beta-blockers*
Timoptic® Ophthalmic / *Beta-blockers*
Timoptic-XE® Ophthalmic / *Beta-blockers*
Tindal® / *Acetophenazine*
TOBI™ Inhalation Solution / *Aminoglycosides*
Tobrex® Ophthalmic / *Aminoglycosides*
Tofranil® / *Imipramine*
Tofranil-PM® / *Imipramine*
Tolectin® / *NSAIDs*
Tolectin® DS / *NSAIDs*
Tolinase® / *Tolazamid*
Topicycline® / *Tetracyclines, topical*
Toposar® / *Chemotherapy drug*
Toprol XL® / *Beta-blockers*
Toradol® Injection / *NSAIDs*
Toradol® / *NSAIDs, oral*
Torecan® / *Thiethylperazine*
Totacillin® / *Penicillins*
Totacillin®-N / *Penicillins*
T-Phyl® / *Theophylline*
Trandate® / *Beta-blockers*
Trendar® (OTC) / *NSAIDs*
Triacet™ / *Corticosteroids*
Triam-A® / *Corticosteroids*
Triam Forte® / *Corticosteroids*
TriCor™ / *Fenofibrate*
Tricosal® / *Choline magnesium trisalicylate*

Triderm® / *Corticosteroids*
Tri-Kort® / *Corticosteroids*
Trilafon® / *Perphenazine*
Tri-Levlen® / *Oral contraceptives*
Trilisate® / *Choline magnesium trisalicylate*
Trilog® / *Corticosteroids*
Trilone® / *Corticosteroids*
Trimox® / *Penicillins*
Trimpex® / *Trimethoprim*
Tri-Norinyl® / *Oral contraceptives*
Triphasil® / *Oral contraceptives*
Tristoject® / *Corticosteroids*
Tritec® / *Ranitidine bismuth citrate*
Trovan™ / *Fluoroquinolones*
Tuinal® / *Barbiturates*

U-Cort™ / *Corticosteroids*
Ultracef® / *Cephalosporins*
Unasyn® / *Penicillins*
Uni-Dur® / *Theophylline*
Unipen® Injection / *Penicillins*
Unipen® Oral / *Penicillins*
Uniphyl® / *Theophyllin*
Uni-Pro® (OTC) / *NSAIDs*
Univasc® / *Moexipril*
Uri-Tet® Oral / *Oxytetracycline*
Urobak® / *Sulfonamides*

Valisone® / *Corticosteroids*
Valium® / *Diazepam*
Vantin® / *Cephalosporins*
Vasotec® / *Enalapril*
Vasotec® IV / *Enalapril*
V-Cillin K® / *Penicillins*
Veban® / *Chemotherapy drug*
Veetids® / *Penicillins*
Velosef® / *Cephalosporins*
Ventolin / *Albuterol*
VePesid® Injection / *Chemotherapy drug*
VePesid® Oral / *Chemotherapy drug*
Verelan® / *Verapamil*
Vibramycin® / *Doxycycline*
Vibramycin® IV / *Doxycycline*

Vibra-Tabs® / *Doxycycline*
Videx® / *Didanosine*
Vincasar® PFS™ Injection / *Chemotherapy drug*
Viramune® / *Nevirapine*
Visken® / *Beta-blockers*
Vistaril® / *Hydroxyzine*
Vivactil® / *Protriptyline*
Volmax / *Albuterol*
Voltaren® Ophthalmic / *NSAIDs*
Voltaren® Oral / *NSAIDs*
Voltaren® Oral -XR / *Oral NSAIDs*

Westcort® / *Corticosteroids*
Winstrol® / *Stanozolol*
Wycillin® / *Penicillins*
Wymox® / *Penicillins*

Xanax® / *Alprazolam*

Yutopar® / *Ritodrine*

Zagam® / *Fluoroquinolones*
Zanosar® / *Chemotherapy drug*
Zantac® / *Ranitidine hydrochloride*
Zantac® 75 (OTC) / *Ranitidine hydrochloride*
Zarontin® / *Ethosuximide*
Zebeta® / *Beta-blockers*
Zerit® / *Stavudine*
Zaroxolyn / *Metoblazone*
Zestril® / *Lisinopril*
Ziagen® / *Abacavir*
Zinacef® Injection / *Cephalosporins*
Zithromax™ / *Macrolides*
Zocor® / *Simvastatin*
Zolicef® / *Cephalosporins*
Zoloft® / *Sertraline*
Zonalon® Topical Cream / *Doxepin*
Zonegran® / *Zonisamide*
ZORprin® / *Aspirin*
Zosyn™ / *Penicillins*
Zovia® / *Oral contraceptives*
Zymenol® (OTC) / *Mineral oil*

GLOSSARY

ACE inhibitors Angiotensin-converting enzyme inhibitors, a class of drugs used to treat high blood pressure.

acetylcholine The primary neurotransmitter involved in thought and memory processes in the brain.

acidosis Abnormal acid condition in the body.

ATP Adenosine triphosphate, the body's primary fuel and energy source.

adrenal cortex Outer layer of the adrenal glands, which secrete steroid hormones.

adrenalin Also called epinephrine, a secretion of the adrenal medulla that stimulates the sympathetic nervous system and causes an increase in the heart rate and blood pressure.

adrenal glands Glands that regulate electrolyte levels, influence metabolism, and respond to stress.

adult-onset diabetes A form of diabetes, also called non-insulin-dependent or Type II diabetes, in which the body produces insulin but does not use it effectively.

aldehydes A form of retinoid that has vitamin A activity.

alpha tocopherol The most common and most potent form of vitamin E.

amino acids Chemical compounds that are the building blocks of various types of protein.

anemia A disorder characterized by lower than normal red blood cell count.

angina Chest pain caused by insufficient supply of oxygen to the heart muscle; a result of coronary artery disease.

anorexia Self-imposed starvation to lose and maintain very low body weight.

anoxia Lack of oxygen in bodily tissues and blood.

antacids Agents used to counteract acidity in the body, which causes indigestion; the two types are those containing magnesium and aluminum salts and those that contain sodium bicarbonate.

antibiotics Drugs administered to combat bacterial infections.

antibodies Disease-fighting proteins created by the immune system in response to specific antigens, forming the basis for immunity.

anticoagulants Agents that slow blood coagulation or clotting and prevent new clots from forming.

anticonvulsants Anti-seizure medications.

antioxidants Disease-fighting nutrients that protect the body from the harmful effects of free radicals.

arrhythmias Irregularities or loss of normal rhythm of the heartbeat.

ascorbic acid Vitamin C; effective in treating viruses.

atherosclerosis Hardening and narrowing of the arteries as a result of build-up of cholesterol plaques, the leading cause of heart disease.

ATP Adenosine triphosphate, a chemical the body uses for immediate energy.

autism A disorder in which a young child does not develop normal social relationships, behaves in compulsive and ritualistic ways, and frequently has poor communication skills.

autoimmune disorders Conditions in which the immune system misreads normal antigens and creates antibodies and directs T cells against the body's own tissues.

basal metabolism Amount of energy the body uses at rest.

beneficial bacteria Microorganisms that promote a healthy intestinal tract, two of which are *Lactobacillus acidophilus* (or *L. acidophilus*) and *bifidobacteria bifidus* (or *bifidus*).

benign prostatic hyperplasia (BPH) Enlargement of the prostate gland that is noncancerous.

benzodiazepines The primary class of anti-anxiety medications.

beriberi The classic disease resulting from a vitamin B_1 deficiency.

beta-blockers Drugs that slow the heartbeat.

beta-carotene The precursor to vitamin A; one of a group of some 500 plant compounds called carotenoids.

biotin One of the B complex vitamins.

blood glucose Sugar carried in the blood.

blood lipids Cholesterol and triglycerides in the blood.

body composition The proportion of fat and nonfat components of the human body.

calciferol Vitamin D, known as the "sunshine vitamin." formed in the body by the action of the sun's ultraviolet rays on the skin, converting the biological precursor into vitamin D.

calcium channel blockers Drugs that reduce the contraction of muscles that squeeze blood vessels; used to treat hypertension, angina, and arrhythmia.

calcium pantothenate Commercial form of Vitamin B_5.

candida A fungus or yeast microorganism that produces toxins in the body.

capillaries The smallest vessels in the circulatory system, connecting the arteries and veins.

carboxylation A chemical reaction in which carbon dioxide is added to acceptor molecules.

cardiac arrhythmias Irregularities or loss of normal rhythm of the heartbeat.

cardiomyopathies Diseases related to the heart muscle.

cardiovascular Pertaining to the heart and blood vessels.

carnitine An amino acid that facilitates the transport of fats across cellular membranes for metabolism and the production of energy.

carotenoids A class of nutrients derived from plants and characterized by their yellow color (carrots, yams, squash, cantaloupe, etc.).

carotenosis Harmless orange coloration of the skin, most noticeable on the palms of the hands and the soles of the feet, resulting from excess intake of beta-carotene.

carpal tunnel syndrome A repetitive motion injury that results from activities involving the hands and wrists such as keyboarding.

cataracts A disease of the eye in which the lens loses its transparency, impairing eyesight.

catecholamines Hormones that include epinephrine and norepinephrine.

CD4 cells Cells that are a part of the immune system, categorized as T killer cells.

celiac disease An immunologic disease process based on intolerance to gluten, affecting the colon. Symptoms include severe abdominal pain and potential life-threatening allergic reactions.

cervical dysplasia Development of abnormal cells in the uterus; considered a pre-cancerous condition.

cfu's Colony-forming units, the measurement for dosages of probiotics.

chelates Mineral substances that are bonded to proteins to improve absorption.

chelosis Cracked corners of the mouth, a symptom of riboflavin deficiency.

cholestasis Bile impairment or blockage.

cholesterol Lipids (fats) that travel in the blood in the form of lipoproteins.

circadian rhythm The normal cycle of biologic functions that occur within a 24-hour period.

cleft lip A congenital defect resulting in a deep fissure of the lip running upward to the nose.

cleft palate An inborn defect that involves the upper lip, hard palate, and/or soft palate.

coagulation Clotting, as in blood clots.

cobalamin Vitamin B_{12}, an essential growth factor that also plays a vital role in the metabolism of all cells, especially those of the intestinal tract, bone marrow, and nervous tissue.

coenzyme A The only known biologically active form of pantothenic acid.

coenzymes Substances that are necessary to drive biochemical reactions in the body.

coenzyme Q_{10} (CoQ_{10}) An important antioxidant and also performs vital roles in generating energy in the mitochondria of all cells.

collagen Fibrous protein material found in skin, bone, cartilage, tendons, and ligaments.

colonocytes The cells that form the inner surface of the colon.

colorectal cancer Cancer of the colon and rectum.

complexing agents Compounds, such as phytates, oxalates, and phosphates, that form insoluble iron complexes and thereby reduce absorption.

congestive heart failure A syndrome in which the heart is unable to pump enough blood to meet the body's needs for oxygen and nutrients; "congestive" refers to the resulting build-up of fluids in the body.

corticosteroids Any of the steroid hormones produced by the adrenal cortex or synthetically.

cortisol A hormone that regulates the metabolism of carbohydrates, fats, and proteins and also has an anti-inflammatory action.

cretinism A severe condition arising in the developing fetus, resulting from iodine deficiency in the mother, and characterized by both mental and physical retardation.

Crohn's disease A chronic autoimmune disorder involving the gastrointestinal tract and most commonly resulting in the scarring and thickening of the walls of the ileum, colon, or both.

cyanocobalamin The most stable and most active form of vitamin B_{12}.

cysteine An amino acid

cytokines Chemical messengers in the body that influence immunologic and inflammatory response.

d-alpha tocopherol Natural vitamin E.

deamination A chemical reaction in which NH_2 groups are removed from certain amino acids in amino acid metabolism.

decarboxylase An enzyme that catalyzes one of the steps in the conversion of tryptophan to serotonin.

decarboxylation A reaction that removes carbon dioxide from molecules in amino acid metabolism.

dehydration Abnormal depletion of body fluids.

dehydrogenases Enzymes that function anaerobically (do not require oxygen).

dementia A slowly progressive decline in mental abilities including memory, thinking, and judgment.

dermatologic Refers to the skin

dermatitis Inflammation of the skin.

desulfuration Transfer of sulfhydro groups in amino acid metabolism.

DHA fatty acid Docosahexanoic acid, an omega-3 fatty acid that is essential for nerve and brain health.

diabetes A group of metabolic diseases characterized by hyperglycemia resulting from defects in insulin secretion, insulin action, or both.

diuretics Agents that increase urine secretion.

DNA (deoxyribonucleic acid) Strings of nucleic acids that affect the growth and repair of all cells and are the molecular basis of heredity.

dopamine A neurotransmitter in the brain that is thought to cause some forms of psychosis and abnormal movement disorders, such as Parkinson's disease.

dysbiosis A digestive condition stemming from toxins produced by unfavorable bacteria in the intestinal tract and characterized by gas and bloating; affects absorption of nutrients and may lead to a variety of other health problems.

dysplasia The abnormal development or growth of cells.

eczema A skin inflammation, sometimes accompanied by itching.

edema Excessive accumulation of fluid that causes swelling.

elastin Fibrous protein material found in skin, bone, cartilage, tendons, and ligaments.

electrolytes The dissociated ions — potassium, sodium, and chloride—responsible for osmotic pressure in body fluids.

endothelial cells Specialized epithelial tissue that lines the inside of the blood and lymph vessels, body cavities, glands, and organs.

enzymes Catalysts that facilitate chemical reactions in the body.

epidemiological Refers to the study of diseases in a population.

epithelial Refers to surface cells of many glands, organs, and skin.

erythrocytes Mature red blood cells, which carry oxygen from the lungs to the tissues and carbon dioxide from the tissues to the lungs.

essential nutrients Vitamins, minerals, amino acids, or fatty acids the body cannot make and must be obtained through the diet.

estrogen A secondary sex hormone.

extracellular fluids Bodily fluids that include the blood, lymph, and the fluid in the spaces between cells.

fatty acids Class of compounds containing long hydrocarbons.

fibrocystic breasts A condition of benign lumps or cyst formation in the breasts, resulting in, for many women, tenderness, pain, increased menstrual flow.

fibrosis Abnormal formation of fibrous tissue.

flavin A vitamin classification of yellow, fluorescent pigments.

flavoprotein Enzymes that function as hydrogen carriers in the electron transport system, resulting in the production of energy within the mitochondria.

fluorosis A mottling discoloration of the teeth that occurs in children if they ingest too much fluoride during tooth development.

folic acid A member of the B vitamin group, a necessary body nutrient.

free radicals Substances formed during metabolism that attack and damage proteins and lipids, leading to the disease.

"friendly" bacteria Microorganisms that promote a healthy intestinal tract, two of which are *Lactobacillus acidophilus* (*L. acidophilus*) and *bifidobacteria bifidus* (or bifidus).

GABA Gamma amino butyric acid, a neurotransmitter in the brain.

gastrointestinal tract The digestive path in the body that consists of the stomach and intestines.

gingivitis Inflammation of the gums, the earliest stage of periodontal disease.

glaucoma A disease of the eye in which the optic nerve is damaged and may cause loss of vision and blindness.

glucose Blood sugar.

glucose tolerance factor (GTF) A form of chromium.

glutathione An antioxidant that improves liver function and detoxification.

glycogen Storage form of glucose in the body.

glycoproteins Protein-sugar complexes necessary for the growth and maintenance of connective tissue and cartilage.

goiter Enlargement of the thyroid gland.

goitrogens Naturally occurring substances in some foods that can inhibit the synthesis and secretion of thyroid hormones.

growth hormone A hormone produced by the pituitary gland that regulates the growth of bone, lean muscle, and other body tissues.

HDL cholesterol High-density cholesterol, the "good" cholesterol.

heart palpitation Pounding or racing of the heart.

hemochromatosis A genetic defect, usually occurring in men, which causes excessive iron absorption and results in damage to the heart, liver, spleen and pancreas.

hemoglobin The oxygen-carrying protein in red blood cells, which contains iron.

hepatitis Inflammation of the liver.

histamines Substances that are produced in response to allergens.

homocysteine An amino acid produced from the metabolism of the essential amino acid methionine that normally exists only briefly; when elevated, a toxic substance that generates inflammation and presents a seriously increased risk for developing atherosclerosis, the leading cause of heart disease.

hormones Products of living cells that circulate in body fluids and produce specific effects on the activity of cells different from their point of origin.

hyaluronidase An enzyme found in malignant tumors.

hyperhomocysteinemia Elevated homocysteine level, now recognized as a serious independent risk factor for cardiovascular disease.

hyperkalemia Potassium toxicity.

hyperthyroidism A condition of excessive thyroid hormones in the blood.

hypocholesterolemia Underactive biosynthesis of cholesterol, which may be associated with manganese deficiency.

hypoglycemia Abnormally low concentration of glucose (sugar) in the blood.

hypogonadism Underdevelopment of sex organs.

hypokalemia Potassium depletion.

HMG-CoA reductase A class of cholesterol-lowering drugs also known as the statins.

hydroxylation The adding of a hydroxyl group in a chemical reaction.

hydroxyapatite A calcium carbonate/calcium phosphate compound that gives bones and teeth rigidity and strength.

hyperbilirubinaemia elevated bilirubin in the body

hypercalcemia A disease of the parathyroid glands characterized by abnormally high concentration of calcium circulating in the blood instead of being stored in the bones; can result from toxic doses of vitamin D.

hyperhomocysteinemia Elevated homocysteine level in the body

hypertension High blood pressure.

hypochlorhydria Low production of hydrochloric acid in the stomach, which impedes iron absorption.

hypothalamus A gland, located in the lower part of the brain, that controls vital body functions.

hypothyroidism Underactive thyroid with symptoms including fatigue, depression, sensitivity to cold, and lower metabolic rate.

hysterectomy Surgical removal of the uterus

ileal Pertaining to the last segment of the small intestine

immune system A major body system that protects the body from harmful substances.

immunity The body's resistance to specific diseases.

inflammation chemistry inhibitors Agents that assist in the regulation of inflammatory processes

inositol A sugar-like, water-soluble member of the B vitamin complex; a component of phospholipids, where it is synthesized in the intestinal tract by the normal or "friendly" bacteria.

insulin A hormone that regulates the transport of glucose to body cells and stimulates the conversion of excess glucose to glycogen for storage.

intracellular fluids Fluids that are found within the cells.

interferon A disease-fighting protein produced by the T cells when invaded by a virus.

interleukin II A cytokine that helps regulate functions in the body.

intrinsic factor A protein in gastric secretions that is necessary for the absorption of vitamin B_{12}.

iodide The form of iodine in the intestinal tract, where it is absorbed and transported to the thyroid gland.

"iodine goiter" Enlargement of the thyroid gland resembling goiter, resulting from chronic excessive intake of iodine.

iron-deficiency anemia A condition in which red blood cells contain less than optimum hemoglobin and consequently carry less oxygen.

I.U. International Units, a system of measurement that applies to some vitamins.

jaundice Yellow discoloration of the skin and other tissues caused by a higher than normal bilirubin level in the blood.

keratin A hard protein that, when it plugs hair follicles, results in a condition called keratinization.

keratinization A condition of dry, scaly, rough skin resulting from a deficiency of Vitamin A.

ketones Products of the breakdown of fats in the body.

killer cells Disease-fighting white blood cells

Krebs cycle Oxidation-reduction reactions involving the production of energy from carbohydrates.

lactose intolerance An allergy to milk and dairy products.

LDL-cholesterol Low density lipoprotein, the "bad" cholesterol, which increases the risk for some forms of cardiovascular disease.

lean body mass Body weight minus body fat.

lecithin A complex phospholipid that is widely distributed in the body.

leukemia A cancer characterized by abnormal concentrations of white blood cells

leukocytes White blood cells.

lipids Blood fats.

lipopolysaccharides Compounds necessary for the growth and maintenance of connective tissue and cartilage.

macrocytic anemia A form of anemia characterized by abnormally enlarged red blood cells.

macrophages A type of T cell that protects the body as part of the immune response.

macular degeneration A progressive disease that results in the loss of central vision but not total blindness and usually affects older people.

malignant melanoma A type of skin cancer.

malnutrition vomiting Vomiting with nutrient depletion.

MAO inhibitors A class of drugs that inhibit the enzyme monoamine oxidase

megaloblastic anemia A form of anemia affecting red blood cells and producing symptoms of tiredness, weakness, diarrhea, and weight loss.

melanin Skin pigment that protects the skin against some of the sun's harmful ultraviolet rays.

melatonin The brain hormone that triggers or induces sleep; secreted by pineal gland

metabolic alkalosis A rare condition caused by a chloride deficiency.

metabolic rate Total amount of energy the body expends in a given amount of time.

metabolism All energy and material transformations that take place within living cells necessary to sustain life.

metabolites Substances produced during metabolism.

metalloenzymes Enzymes that utilize trace minerals for function.

methionine An essential amino acid that is converted by folic acid from homocysteine and produces SAMe.

microflora Tiny plant life that lives in the body, some beneficial and some not.

micronutrients Nutrients the body requires in small amounts.

mineralization Formation of bone.

mitochondria A component of cells that produces all energy necessary for cell function.

mitochondrial antioxidant A compound that protects against the toxic superoxide dismutase effects of oxygen during energy production.

mitral valve prolapse Abnormal protrusion of the mitral valve of the heart that results in incomplete closure of the valve.

mucopolysaccharides Sugars necessary for the growth and maintenance of connective tissue and cartilage.

myelin Tissue that covers and insulates nerves and is essential to the functioning and maintenance of the nervous system.

myoglobin An iron-containing protein in muscles that accepts oxygen and serves as an oxygen storage reservoir.

myoinositol The metabolically active form of inositol, which occurs abundantly in muscle tissue.

myxedema Lowered function of the thyroid gland caused by iodine deficiency.

neural tube defects Birth defect due to folic acid deficiency.

neurologic Pertaining to the nerves or nervous system.

neuropeptides Proteins that are involved in neurologic (nerve) function.

neurotransmitters Chemical messengers that transmit messages between nerve cells.

nitrosamines Carcinogens that are produced by the body or taken in from the diet.

norepinephrine A hormone that stimulates the sympathetic nervous system and is produced in the adrenal medulla.

nucleic acids DNA and RNA.

Neutrophilic Hypersegmentation Index (NHI) A laboratory test used to identify folic acid insufficiency.

niacin Vitamin B_3

niacin flush A vasodilation reaction resulting in redness of the skin and itching, which typically occurs if dosages of niacin exceed 50mg at a time.

noradrenalin A hormone that stimulates the sympathetic nervous system; also known as norepinephrine.

nyctalopia Night blindness.

nystagmus An involuntary, constant movement of the eyeball.

ophthalmologists Physicians specializing in diagnosing and treating diseases and disorders of the eye.

osteoarthritis A form of arthritis commonly associated with aging.

osteoblasts Essential substance for normal bone growth and development, influenced by the nutrient manganese.

osteoclasts Substances that stimulates the break down of bone (clast = break down).

osteoarthritis The most common form of arthritis, affecting primarily the hands and weight-bearing joints.

osteocalcin A protein in bone that attracts calcium to bone tissue.

osteomalacia Gradual softening and bending of the bones with varying severity of pain.

osteoporosis A disease condition characterized by porous, brittle bones that break easily.

OTC Abbreviation for over-the-counter; nonprescription drugs.

oxidases Enzymes that function aerobically (utilize oxygen).

pagophagia Deliberately consuming large quantities of ice, related to iron deficiency.

palpitation A pounding or racing heart.

pancreas An organ that secretes digestive juices and enzymes into the small intestine.

pantotheine A sulfur-containing compound derived from pantothenic acid .

pantothenic acid Vitamin B_5, so named by its discoverer, Roger Willliams, because it is present in all body cells.

para-aminosalicylic acid An anti-tubercular agent often administered with isoniazid.

parathyroid gland A gland that regulates calcium levels in the body.

Parkinson's disease A chronic, progressive, degenerative disorder of the central nervous system that affects muscular control.

pathological Pertaining to disease.

pellagra Severe deficiency of niacin, which means "rough skin; additional symptoms are dementia and diarrhea.

periodontal disease A condition affecting the gums of the mouth.

peripheral neuropathy A condition of the nerves characterized by numbness, tingling, or a burning sensation.

permeability Capable of being penetrated by liquids or gases.

pernicious anemia An autoimmune disorder that results from either inadequate vitamin B_{12} intake or reduced gastric (stomach) secretion of intrinsic factor.

peroxidase One of the most important antioxidant enzymes in the immune system.

pharmacologic dose Amounts of a drug known to have a physiologic effect.

phosphatidyl choline (PC) A substance that promotes flexibility in cellular membranes.

phosphatidylinositol Part of phospholipids in cellular membranes; helps to mediate cellular responses to external stimuli and facilitates the production of arachidonic acid.

phosphate An organic compound needed by the body.

phosphodiesterase inhibitor A substance that produces the same action as some asthma medications.

phospholipids A type of lipid containing two fatty acids and a phosphate group.

photophobia Eye sensitivity or pain resulting from bright light.

phytic acid Form of inositol found in plants.

pineal gland A gland located in the brain that secretes melatonin, which influences the sleep/wakefulness cycle.

pituitary gland The gland that directs the activity of the other endocrine glands.

plaque Build-up of fatty acids in the blood vessels, which can restrict blood flow.

platelets The smallest elements of the blood.

polyamines A group of compounds, consisting of spermidine, puescine, and spermine, essential for cellular growth and differentiation, gene expression, protein phosphorylation, neuron regeneration, and the repair of DNA.

polyunsaturated fatty acids Fatty acids that do not have full saturation of hydrogen in their chemical structure.

PMS Premenstrual syndrome; a result of increased estrogen production, which could cause symptoms such as heavy menstrual flow, tender breasts, irregular bleeding, and emotional mood swings.

postural hypotension Low blood pressure when changing from a lying or sitting position to a standing position.

probiotics Beneficial bacteria in the gastrointestinal tract.

prostaglandins Hormone-like chemicals that regulate cellular activities.

proteins Complex organic compounds formed by combinations of amino acids; used in the body to build and repair tissues and are part of hormones, antibodies, and enzymes.

prothrombin A substance necessary for normal clotting of blood.

provitamin A A precursor of vitamin A in fruits and vegetables, consisting of two molecules of vitamin A linked together.

psoriasis A chronic autoimmune disorder of the skin.

pyridoxal phosphate (PLP) Active form of vitamin B_6

pyridoxine Vitamin B_6

quinines Vitamin K groups: (a) phylloquinone (K1), which occurs in green plants; (b) menaquinone (K2), synthesized by intestinal bacteria; and (c) menadione (K3), manufactured synthetically.

RDA Recommended Dietary Allowance, standards for daily intake of nutrients for healthy people, set by the National Academy of Sciences.

R.E. Retinol equivalents, used to measure dosages of vitamin A and beta-carotene.

renal tubular acidosis A condition characterized by too much acid in the body resulting from a defect in kidney function.

retinoids A class of compounds that include vitamin A and occur only in animal products.

rickets A demineralized bone disease caused by calcium and vitamin D deficiencies in early childhood.

riboflavin Vitamin B_2, a member of a group of yellow fluorescent pigments called flavins.

RNA Ribonucleic acid, the genetic material involved in formation of cell proteins.

SAMe S-adenosyl methionine, a metabolite of the essential amino acid and a co-factor in three important biochemical pathways.

schizophrenia Psychotic disorder characterized by delusions, hallucinations, disorganized or incoherent speech, and disruptive behavior.

scurvy Nutritional deficiency disease deriving from insufficiency of vitamin C.

seborrheic dermatitis A condition of dry, itchy, scaly skin that can result from a deficiency of riboflavin or pyridoxine.

serotonin A neurotransmitter that, when released in the brain in the form of melatonin,, has a role in sleep and also elevates the mood.

serum cholesterol Cholesterol in the blood, as contrasted with dietary cholesterol.

silicosis An occupational lung disease caused by inhalation of silicon dioxide dust.

sodium ascorbate A form of vitamin C.

soluble Capability of dissolving in water (water-soluble) or fat (fat-soluble); the nutrients are classified into either of these two groups.

spina bifida An inborn defect in which the spinal canal doesn't close around the spinal cord and leaves it exposed.

spooning Inversion of the nail bed that produces an effect that looks like a spoon.

statins A class of cholesterol-lowering drugs also known as HMG-CoA reductase inhibitors.

sulfite oxidase enzyme responsible for breakdown of sulfur bearing amino acids.

sulfolipids Sulfur-containing lipids, or body fats.

tachycardia An abnormally fast heartbeat.

tardive dyskinesia Side effect after long-term drug regimen, characterized by distortion or impairment of voluntary movement as in a tic or spasm.

T lymphocytes White blood cells that circulate to fight invading organisms as part of the immune response.

testosterone Secondary sex hormone.

tetany Muscle spasms.

tetrahydrofolic acid (THFA) The biologically active form of folic acid.

thiamin Vitamin B$_1$

thrombus Blood clot

thymus A ductless (endocrine) gland that plays a major rule in the immune system.

thyroglobulin Storage form of iodine in the thyroid gland.

thyroid gland A gland that regulates the body's metabolism and is influenced by the amount of iodine ingested.

thyroxin The principal hormone of the thyroid gland.

T-lymphocytes Specialized white blood cells that identify pathogens and help to fight pathogens.

tocopherols Vitamin E.

total parenteral nutrition (TPN) Nutrition administered intravenously.

toxins Poisonous substances that are the product of metabolic activity and are capable of inducing the production of antibodies within the body.

trace minerals Minerals that the body requires in very small amounts.

transamination Transfer of amino groups in amino acid metabolism.

transsulfuration The synthesis of cysteine, glutathione, and taurine.

TRH Thyroid-releasing hormone.

triglycerides Fatty substances used for energy or stored by muscle or fat cells.

tryptophan An amino acid that is the precursor of niacin.

TSH Thyroid-stimulating hormone.

Type II diabetes A form of diabetes, also called non-insulin-dependent or adult-onset diabetes, in which the body produces insulin but does not use it effectively.

ubiquinone Another term for coenzyme Q$_{10}$.

ulcerative colitis an inflammatory condition of the colon that destructs the colon lining in the large intestine and the rectum.

uric acid a breakdown product of protein metabolism.

vascular Refers to blood vessels.

vascular endothelial cells Cells in the tissue lining the internal walls of blood vessels.

vasodilation Dilation of the vascular tissue, enhancing circulation.

vitamin K A nutrient that regulates blood-clotting mechanisms and calcium deposition into the bone matrix.

Wernicke–Korsakoff syndrome A condition of severe deficiency associated with alcohol consumption, with symptoms ranging from mild confusion to severely impaired memory and cognitive function, and coma.

xanthine oxidase An enzyme from cow's milk.

xeropthalmia Drying and hardening of the membranes that line the eyes.

APPENDIX: SCIENTIFIC BASIS FOR GENERIC DRUGS

This appendix provides the scientific basis for generic drugs included in this reference guide and the nutrients they deplete, according to the following designations:

SB1: The most common rationale for including a drug in this book; indicates that the scientific studies reporting a nutrient depletion(s) were conducted using this specific drug.

SB2: Indicate that studies from drugs in the same pharmacological class have reported nutrient depletions. For example, assume that no studies have reported that drug X has depleted any nutrients. Nevertheless, if studies have reported that other drugs in the same pharmacological class have caused nutrient depletions, it can be assumed that drug X could deplete the same nutrients.

SB3: Refers to a drug that works the same way as another drug that is known to cause a nutrient depletion (both drugs have the same mechanism of action.)

SB4: Designates drugs for which there is inferred or indirect evidence of depletion based on disruption of physiological processes. An example is when chemotherapy drugs or antibiotics disrupt the normal functioning of the gastrointestinal tract.

Drug	SB	Depletes
acetohexamide	SB1	coenzyme Q10
acetophenazine	SB2	vitamin B_2
albuterol	SB1	potassium
alprazolam	SB1	melatonin
aluminum hydroxide	SB1	calcium, phosphorus
aluminum hydroxide and magnesium salts	SB2	calcium, phosphorus, folic acid
aluminum hydroxide, magnesium hydroxide, and simethicone	SB2	calcium, phosphorus, folic acid

Drug	SB	Depletes
aminoglycosides	SB4	bifidobacteria bifidum, biotin, inositol, lactobacillus acidophilus, vitamin B_1, vitamin B_2, vitamin B_3, vitamin B_6, vitamin B_{12}, vitamin K
amitriptyline	SB1	coenzyme Q_{10}, vitamin B_2
amoxapine	SB2	coenzyme Q_{10}, vitamin B_2
amphotericin B	SB1	calcium, magnesium, potassium, sodium
aspirin	SB1	folic acid, iron, potassium, sodium, vitamin C, calcium, vitamin B
atenolool	SB1	melatonin
atorvastatin	SB2	coenzyme Q_{10}
barbiturates	SB1	biotin, calcium, folic acid, vitamin D, vitamin K
benazepril	SB2	zinc
benzthiazide	SB2	coenzyme Q_{10}, magnesium, potassium, zinc
beta-blockers	SB1	coenzyme Q_{10}
bisacodyl	SB1	depletes potassium
bumetanide	SB2	calcium, magnesium, potassium, vitamin B_1, vitamin B_6, vitamin C, zinc
captopril	SB1	zinc
carbamazepine	SB1	biotin, folic acid, vitamin D
cephalosporins	SB4	bifidobacteria bifidum, biotin, inositol, lactobacillus acidophilus, vitamin B_1, vitamin B_2, vitamin B_3, vitamin B_6, vitamin B_{12}, vitamin K
cerivastatin	SB2	coenzyme Q_{10}
chloropromazine	SB1	coenzyme Q_{10}, melatonin, vitamin B_2
chlorothiazide	SB2	coenzyme Q_{10}, magnesium, potassium, sodium, zinc
chlorotrianisene	SB2	magnesium, vitamin B_{12}
chlortetracycline	SB2	biotin, calcium, inositol, iron, magnesium, vitamin B_1, vitamin B_2, vitamin B_3, vitamin B_6, vitamin B_{12}, vitamin K
	SB4	bifidobacteria bifidum (bifidus), lactobacillus acidophilus
chlorthalidone	SB1	zinc
cholestyramine resin	SB1	beta-carotene, calcium, folic acid, iron, magnesium, phosphorus, vitamin A, vitamin B_{12}, vitamin D, vitamin E, vitamin K, zinc
choline magnesium trisalicylate	SB2	folic acid, iron, potassium, sodium, vitamin C
choline salicylate	SB2	folic acid, iron, potassium, sodium, vitamin C
cimetidine	SB1	calcium, folic acid, iron, vitamin B, vitamin D, zinc

Drug	SB	Depletes
clofibrate	SB1	copper, vitamin B_{12}, vitamin E, zinc
clomipramine	SB2	coenzyme Q_{10}, vitamin B_2
clonidine	SB1	coenzyme Q_{10}
colchicines	SB1	beta-carotene, potassium, sodium, vitamin B_{12}, calcium, phosphorus
colestipol	SB1	beta-carotene, folic acid, iron, vitamin A, vitamin B_{12}, vitamin D, vitamin E
corticosteroids	SB1	calcium, folic acid, magnesium, potassium, selenium, vitamin C, vitamin D, zinc; also chromium, vitamin A
co-trimoxazole	SB1	folic acid
	SB4	bifidobacteria bifidum (bifidus), lactobacillus acidophilus
delavirdine	SB2	carnitine, copper, vitamin B_{12}, zinc
demeclocycline	SB2	biotin, calcium, inositol, iron, magnesium, vitamin B_1, vitamin B_2, vitamin B_3, vitamin B_6, vitamin B_{12}, vitamin K
	SB4	bifidobacteria bifidum (biridus), lactobacillus acidophilus
desipramine	SB2	coenzyme Q_{10}, vitamin B_2
diazepam	SB1	melatonin
didanosine	SB2	carnitine, copper, vitamin B_{12}, zinc
diethylstilbestrol	SB2	magnesium, vitamin B_6
digoxin	SB1	calcium, magnesium, phosphorus, vitamin B_1
doxepin	SB2	coenzyme Q_{10}, vitamin B_2
doxycycline	SB2	biotin, calcium, inositol, iron, magnesium, vitamin B_1, vitamin B_2, virtamin B_3, vitamin B_6, vitamin B_{12}, vitamin K
	SB4	bifidobacteria bifidum (bifidus, lactobacillus acidophilus
EDTA	SB1	calcium
enalapril	SB1	zinc
estrogen	SB2	magnesium, vitamin B_6, niacin
estrogens, conjugated	SB1	magnesium, vitamin B_6, niacin
estrogens, esterified	SB2	magnesium, vitamin B_6, niacin
ethacrynic acid	SB3	calcium, magnesium, potassium, vitamin B_1, vitamin B_6, vitamin C, zinc
ethambutol	SB1	copper, zinc
famotidine	SB2	calcium, folic acid, iron, vitamin B_{12}, vitamin D, zinc
fenofibrate	SB2	copper, vitamin B_{12}, vitamin E, zinc
Fleet® phosphate enema	SB1	calcium, magnesium

Drug	SB	Depletes
fluoroquinolones	SB4	bifidobacteria bifidum (bifidus), biotin, inositol, lactobacillus acidophilus, vitamin B_1, vitamin B_2, vitamin B_3, vitamin B_6, vitamin B_{12}, vitamin K
fluphenazine	SB2	vitamin B_2
fluvastin	SB2	coenzyme Q_{10}
foscarnet	SB1	calcium, magnesium, potassium
fosinopril	SB2	zinc
fosphenytoin	SB1	calcium, folic acid, vitamin D, vitamin K
furosemide	SB1	calcium, magnesium, potassium, vitamin B_1, vitamin B_6, vitamin C, zinc
gemfibrozil	SB1	coenzyme Q_{10}, vitamin E
glyburide	SB1	coenzyme Q_{10}
haloperidol	SB1	coenzyme Q_{10}, melatonin, vitamin E
hydralazine	SB1	coenzyme Q_{10}, vitamin B_6
hydralazine and hydrochlorothiazide	SB1	coenzyme Q_{10}, vitamin B6, magnesium, potassium, sodium, zinc
hydralazine, hydrochlorothiazide, and reserpine	SB 1	coenzyme Q_{10}, vitamin B6, magnesium, potassium, sodium, zinc
hydrochlorothiazide triamterene	SB1	coenzyme Q_{10}, magnesium, potassium, sodium, zinc
hydrochlorothiazide and triamterene	SB1	calcium, coenzyme Q_{10}, folic acid, magnesium, potassium, sodium, zinc
hydroflumethiazide	SB2	coenzyme Q_{10}, magnesium, potassium, sodium, zinc
hydroxyzine	SB1	melatonin
imipramine	SB1	coenzyme Q_{10}, vitamin B_2
indapamide	SB3	coenzyme $Q_{10,}$ magnesium, potassium, sodium, zinc
indomethacin	SB1	folic acid, iron
isoniazid	SB1	vitamin B_3, vitamin B_6, vitamin D
lamivudine	SB2	carnitine, copper, vitamin B_{12}, zinc
lansoprazole	SB2	vitamin B_{12}
levodopa	SB1	potassium, SAMe, vitamin B_6
levothyroxine	SB1	iron
lisinopril	SB2	zinc
lithium	SB1	inositol
lovastatin	SB1	coenzyme Q_{10}
macrolides	SB4	bifidobacteria bificum, biotin, inositol, lactobacillus acidophilus, vitamin B_1, vitamin B_2, vitamin B_3, vitamin B_6, vitamin B_{12}, vitamin K
magnesium oxide	SB2	calcium, phosphorus
magnesium sulfate	SB2	calcium, phosphorus

Drug	SB	Depletes
mesoridazine	SB2	coenzyme Q_{10}, vitamin B_2
metformin	SB2	coenzyme Q_{10}, folic acid, vitamin B_{12}
methdilazine	SB2	vitamin B_2
methotrexate	SB1	folic acid
methotrimeprazine	SB2	vitamin B_2
methclothiazide	SB2	coenzyme Q_{10}, potassium, zinc
methyldopa	SB1	coenzyme Q_{10}
metolazone	SB3	coenzyme Q_{10}, magnesium, potassium, zinc
metoprolol	SB1	melanin
mineral oil	SB1	beta-carotene, calcium, vitamin A, vitamin D, vitamin E, vitamin K
moexipril	SB2	zinc
neomycin	SB1	beta-carotene, iron, vitamin A, vitamin B_{12}
nevirapine	SB2	carnitine, copper, vitamin B_{12}, zinc
nizatidine	SB2	calcium, folic acid, iron, vitamin B_{12}, vitamin D, zinc
nortriptyline	SB2	coenzyme Q_{10}, vitamin B_2
NSAIDs	SB1	folic acid
omeprazole	SB1	vitamin B_{12}
oral contraceptives	SB1	folic acid, magnesium, vitamin B_2, vitamin B_3, vitamin B_6, vitamin B_{12}, vitamin C, zinc; also selenium, vitamin B_1
oxytetracycline	SB2	bifidus, biotin, calcium, inositol, iron, lactobacillus acidophilus, magnesium, vitamin B_1, vitamin B_2, vitamin B_3, vitamin B_6, vitamin B_{12}, vitamin K
penicillamine	SB1	copper, magnesium, vitamin B_6; also iron
penicillins	SB4	bifidus, biotin, inositol, lactobacillus acidophilus, vitamin B_1, vitamin B_2, vitamin B_3, vitamin B_6, vitamin B_{12} vitamin K
	SB1	potassium
pentamidine	SB4	magnesium
perphenazine	SB2	coenzyme Q_1, vitamin B_2
phenelzine	SB1	vitamin B_6
phenobarbitol	SB1	biotin, calcium, folic acid, vitamin D, vitamin K
phenytoin	SB2	biotin, calcium, folic acid, vitamin B_1, vitamin B_{12}, vitamin D, vitamin K
polythiazide	SB2	coenzyme Q_{10}, magnesium, potassium, zinc
potassium chloride	SB1	vitamin B_{12}
prevastin	SB1	coenzyme Q_{10}
primidone	SB1	biotin, folic acid
prochlorperazine	SB2	coenzyme Q_{10}, vitamin B_2
promazine	SB2	coenzyme Q_{10}, vitamin B_2

Drug	SB	Depletes
promethazine	SB2	coenzyme Q_{10}, vitamin B_2
propranolol	SB1	melatonin
protriptyline	SB2	coenzyme Q_{10}, vitamin B_2
quinesterol	SB2	magnesium, vitamin B_6
quinethazone	SB2	coenzyme Q_{10}, magnesium, potassium, zinc
ramipril	SB2	zinc
rantidine hydrochloride	SB1	calcium, folic acid, iron, vitamin B_{12}, vitamin D, zinc
rifampin	SB1	vitamin D
ritodrine	SB1	potassium
salsalate	SB3	folic acid
simvastatin	SB1	coenzyme Q_{10}
sodium bicarbonate	SB1	potassium, folic acid
stanozolol	SB1	iron
stavudine	SB2	carnitine, copper, vitamin B_{12}, zinc
sulfasalazine	SB1	folic acid
sulfonamides	SB2 or SB4	bifidus, biotink inositol, lactobacillus, acidophilus, vitamin B_1, vitamin B_2, vitamin B_3, vitamin B_6, vitamin B_{12}, vitamin K
terbutaline	SB1	potassium
tetracyclines	SB1	bifidus, biotin, calcium, inositol, iron, lactobacillus acidophilus, magnesium, vitamin B_1, vitamin B_2, vitamin B_3, vitamin B_6, vitamin B_{12}, vitamin K, zinc
theophylline	SB1	vitamin B_6
thiethylperazine	SB2	coenzyme Q_{10}, vitamin B_2
thioridazine	SB2	coenzyme Q_{10}, vitamin B_2
tolazamide	SB1	coenzyme Q_{10}
torsemide	SB2	calcium, magnesium, potassium, vitamin B_1, vitamin B_6, vitamin C, zinc
trandolapril	SB2	zinc
triamterene	SB1	calcium, folic acid, zinc
trichlormethiazide	SB2	magnesium, potassium
trifluoperazine	SB2	coenzyme Q_{10}, vitamin B_2
trimethoprim	SB1 & SB4	biotin, folic acid, inositol, vitamin B_1, vitamin B_2, vitamin B_3, vitamin B_6, vitamin B_{12}, vitamin K
trimipramine	SB2	coenzyme Q_{10}, vitamin B_2
valproic acid	SB1	carnitine, copper, folic acid, selenium, zinc
verapamil	SB1	potassium
zalcitabine	SB2	carnitine, copper, vitamin B_{12}, zinc
zidovudine	SB1	carnitine, copper, vitamin B_{12}, zinc

INDEX

abacavir, 106
acebutolol, 14, 104
ACE inhibitors, 14, 58, 121, 138
acetaldehyde, 150
acetazolamide, 138
acetohexamine, 9, 104
acetophenazine, 46
acetylcholine, 100, 145, 150, 153
acid/alkaline pH balance, 100, 130, 132, 138
acidophilus bifidus, 91, 92, 119
acidosis, 99, 131
acne, 29, 34, 166, 167
adenosine triphosphate (ATP), 105
adrenal cortex/glands, 99, 131, 132, 150, 156
adrenalin, 157
adriamycin, 105, 135
advicor, 104
aging process, xii, 125, 133, 136, 157
agitation, 155
AIDS patients, 56, 167
albuterol, 13
alcohol
  abuse and alcoholism, 118, 121, 130, 144,
    145, 147
  detoxification, 150, 166
  and vitamin deficiencies, 153, 157
  and zinc deficiency, 166
aldehyde oxidase, 127
alkalosis, metabolic, 99
alpha tocopherol, 161–163
alprazolam, 12, 125
aluminum antacids/salts, 4, 26, 110, 130
aluminum hydroxide-containing products, 95
Alzheimer's disease, 101
American Association of Poison Control
  Centers, xi
American Dental Association, 108
amiloride, 104, 110
amino acids, 98, 116, 123, 127, 132, 133,
  139, 140, 153. *See also* protein
aminoglycosides, 5, 33, 91, 92, 95, 113,
  118, 120, 131, 138, 144, 146, 148, 151,
  154, 164
amitriptyline, 21, 104, 146
amlodipine, 15
amoxapine, 104, 146
amphotericin B, 9, 48, 95, 120, 131. 138
anabolic steroids, 22, 79–80

anemia, 26, 111, 152, 157
  macrocytic, 155
  nutrient deficiencies and, 32, 106, 116–117,
    254, 155, 162
  pernicious, 154, 155
angina and CoQ$_{10}$ deficiency, 105
anorexia, 26, 93, 111, 143, 145, 166
anoxia, 133
antacids, 4, 26, 117
  aluminum-containing, 130
  magnesium/aluminum hydroxide, 4, 26
  sodium bicarbonate antacids, 4, 26–27
anti-anxiety agents: benzoediazepines, 4, 27
anti-arthritic medications, 49
antibiotics, 6–7, 27–29, 35, 91, 119
antibodies, 158
anticoagulant drugs, 163
anticonvulsants, 6–8, 35, 134
antidepressants, 134
antidiabetic drugs, 8–9, 46–48
antifungal drugs, 9, 48
antihistamines, 9, 48–49, 158
anti-inflammatory
  drugs, 10–11, 49
  properties of selenium, 135
antimalarial antibiotics, 5, 33
antioxidants, xii, 27, 90, 105, 124, 125–126,
  127, 133, 134, 135, 147, 157, 158, 162
anti-Parkinson's disease drugs, 11, 54
anti-protozoal drugs, 11, 55
antiviral agents, 12, 55
anxiety, 26, 102, 121
anxiolytic drugs, 4. *See also* anti-anxiety
appetite, loss of/poor, and nutrient depletion,
  99, 121, 138, 155, 157
arachidonic acid, 113
arthritis, 107, 109, 153, 167
ascorbic acid, 156–159
aspirin, 10, 52, 95, 110, 116, 131, 138, 150, 156
asthma, 122, 155, 158
atenolol, 14, 58, 104, 125
atherosclerosis, 97, 105, 109, 112, 121, 137,
  152, 153, 158, 162
atorvastin, 104
atovastatin, 17
ATP, 130, 145, 147
autistic infants, 153
avacavir, 98

baby boomers, xi
bacteria, beneficial/"friendly," 27, 28, 29, 34, 35, 91, 92, 93, 112, 113, 118–120
barbiturates, 7, 35, 37, 92, 95, 110, 159, 164
basal metabolism, 115
benazepril, 165
benign prostatic hyperplasia (BPH), 162, 167
benzthiazide, 104, 120, 131, 165
benzodiazepines, 4, 27, 149
beriberi, 144
beta$_2$ adrenergic agonists, 13, 57
beta-blockers, 14, 58, 104, 105
beta-carotene, 90–91, 142, 144
betaine, 101
bifidobacteria bifidus, 4, 28, 91–92
biguanides, 8–9, 46–48
bile acid and sequestrants, 17, 66–67, 150
biotin, 38, 41, 43, 92–93, 139, 140
birth defects
    antacids and, 26
    folic acid and, 32, 37, 111
    vanadium and, 142
    zinc and, 166
bisacodyl, 20, 76–77, 131
bloating/gas, 91, 119
blood cholesterol, 141. *See also* cholesterol
blood clots and blood-clotting, 37, 73, 96, 124, 155, 163, 164
blood lipids, 98, 141
blood pressure, 96, 138, 139, 105. *See also* hypertension
blood sugar regulation, 102, 103, 116
body composition, 103
bone health and bone density, 124, 137, 141, 166
    mineral role in, 94, 96, 97, 108–109, 120, 122
    vitamin role in, 90, 142, 143, 160
boron, 94–95
bowed legs, 160
bowel tolerance, vitamin C and, 159
brain
    vitamin C and, 157
    hormones, 27, 29, 30, 57, 74
breathing, labored, 132
brittle nails, 117
bronchial squamous metaplasia, 112
bronchodilators, 13, 56
bruising, easy, 29, 155, 157, 162
bumetanide, 16, 95, 120, 131, 144, 151, 156, 165
butyrophenones, 22
B vitamins, 4, 92, 111, 113, 119, 144, 146, 148, 150, 151

cadmium, 135
caffeine, 131
calciferol. *See* vitamin D
calcification, 164

calcium, 29, 94, 95–97, 130
    absorption and vitamin D, 30, 33, 36, 38
    depletion as drug effect, 26, 31, 34
    metabolism, 94, 96, 122
    phosphate, 130
    supplementation, 38
    vitamin D and, 161
calcium antagonists, plain, 59
calcium channel blockers, 15, 59–60, 121
calcium citrate, 97
calcium pantothenate, 150
calcium phosphate, 37, 40, 43
cancer
    beta-carotene and, 90
    breast, 106
    chemotherapy, 13, 83
    colorectal, 97
    fluoride and, 108
    folic acid and, 26, 111, 112
    melatonin and, 125
    nickel and, 129
    selenium and, 134, 135
    vitamin A and, 142, 143
    vitamin B$_{12}$ and, 155
    vitamin C and, 157–158
    vitamin D and, 161
    vitamin E and, 163
    vitamin K and, 164
    zinc and, 166
candida yeast organisms, 29
captopril, 14, 165
carbamazepine, 6–7, 41–43, 92, 95, 110, 159
carbohydrates. *See* metabolism
carbon dioxide, transport and excretion of, 138, 166
carboxylation reactions, 93
cardiac glycosides, 15, 59–60
cardiac rhythm/arrhythmias, 105, 132
cardiomyopathies, 135
cardiovascular drugs, 14–16
cardiovascular system and diseases
    chromium and, 102
    coenzyme Q$_{10}$ to treat, 104, 105, 106
    copper role in, 106, 107, 112, 119
    as isoniazid effect, 30
    magnesium and, 121, 122
    selenium and, 135
    silicon and, 137
    vitamin B$_1$ and, 145
    vitamin B$_6$ and, 30, 152
    vitamin C and, 158
    vitamin E and, 162
carnitine, 98–99, 117
carotenoids, 90
carotenosis, 90
carpal tunnel syndrome, 153
catecholamines, 133
celiac disease, 130, 145, 166
centrally acting antihypertensives, 15, 60–61

cephalosporins, 91, 92, 113, 118, 144, 146, 148, 151, 154, 164
cerivastatin, 17, 104
ceruloplasmin, 106
cervical dysplasia, 26, 32, 111, 112, 157
chelosis, 146
chemotherapy drugs, 13, 65–66
chloride, 99–100
chlorpromazine, 21, 104, 125, 146
chlorothiazide (HCTZ), 16, 120, 131, 165
chlorotrianisene, 120, 154
chlorthalidone, 16, 120, 165
choestipol, 116
cholestasis, 134
cholesterol, blood, 102, 103, 107, 119, 123, 133, 149, 150
cholesterol-lowering drugs, 17–18, 66–68
cholestyramine, 17, 67, 90, 95, 110, 116, 120, 142, 154, 159, 161, 164, 165
choline, 100
choline magnesium trisalicylate, 110, 116, 131, 138, 156
choline salicylate, 110, 116, 131, 138, 156
chondroitin sulfate, 139, 140
chromium, 102–103
cimetidine, 23, 95, 110, 116, 154, 159, 165
circadian rhythm, 125
clofibrate, 18, 67, 106, 154, 161, 165
clomipramine, 104, 146
clonidine, 15, 60, 104
cobalamin, 154
cobalt, 154
coenzyme A, 140, 150
coenzyme Q_{10}, 104–106
colchicines, 20, 75–76, 90, 95, 131, 138, 154
colestipol, 17, 67, 90, 110, 142, 154, 159, 161
coloncytes, 92
collagen, 107, 118, 123, 137, 140, 157, 158
common cold, 158
concentration, poor, 138
confusion, 34, 121, 155
congestive heart failure, 105
constipation, 34, 91, 131
cooking, vitamin loss in, 36, 41, 111, 145, 147, 153, 162
copper, 106–108, 126, 167
copper chelates, 107
corticosteroids, 10, 49–52, 95, 110, 120, 131, 134, 142, 156, 157, 159, 165
cortisol, 157
co-trimoxazole, 91, 110, 118, 154
cow's milk, 97, 135, 157
COX-2 inhibitors, 54, 110
cretism, 115
Crohn's disease, 130, 166
cyanocobalamin, 154–156
cycloserine, 5–6, 31–33, 95, 110, 120, 148
cysteine and, 133, 139, 140
cytokines, 134

Dam, Henrik, 164
deamination reactions, 93, 153
decarboxylation, 153
dehydration, 138
dehydrogenases, 147
delavirdine, 98, 106
delusions, 155
dementia, 124, 148, 155
dental cavities, 108, 109
depletion, drug-induced nutrient, vii, ix
depression
    as antacid effect, 26
    biotin deficiency and, 93
    and folic acid deficiency, 111
    inositol and, 113
    magnesium deficiency and, 121
    SAME and 133
    vitamin B_1 and, 145
    vitamin B_2 and, 147
    vitamin B_6 and, 29, 151, 153
    vitamin B_{12} and, 155
    zinc and, 166
dermatitis and dermatologic changes, 93, 147, 148, 151, 152, 155. See also skin
desipramine, 21, 104, 146
desulfuration, 153
detoxification
    alcohol, 150
    liver, 133, 134
    metabolic, of sulfuric acid, 140
dexamethasone, 10
DHA, 41, 42
diabetes, 78
    adult onset (Type II), 102, 103, 121
    and biotin deficiency, 93
    copper and, 107
    magnesium and, 121
    vanadium and, 141
    zinc and, 166
diabetic acidosis, 131
diabetic neuropathy, 113
diarrhea
    as drug effect, 26
    and intestinal bacteria, 91
    nutrient deficiency and, 99, 111, 117, 122, 131, 138, 143, 145, 148, 151, 159, 167
diazepam, 4, 12, 27, 125
diclofenac, 110
didanosine, 98, 106
diethylstilbesterol, 120, 151
diflunisal, 110
digestion, poor, and nutrient depletion, 99. See also bacteria
digoxin, 15, 59–60, 95, 120
diltiazem, 15
diuretics, 99, 105, 145
    loop, 16, 63, 138
    potassium-sparing, 16, 63
    thiazide, 16, 65

disulfide, 140
Diuril, 104
dizziness, 34, 131, 155, 167
DNA, 36, 39, 41, 43, 47, 63, 111, 112, 120, 130, 133, 155, 155, 167
dopamine, 118, 124
dosepaks, 49
doxepin, 21, 104, 146
drowsiness, 167
dysbiosis, 91, 92, 119, 120
dysplasia, 112

eczema, 129, 147, 162, 167
edema, 34, 131, 139, 145
EDTA, 24, 85, 95
elanapril, 14, 165
elastin, 107, 118, 158
elderly
    vitamin B_{12} and, 35, 155
    vitamin C and, 157
    vitamin D and, 160
electrolytes, 18, 99, 100, 131, 138
energy level, and nutrient depletion, 98, 102, 105
energy production, 105, 150, 153, 157, 166
enoxacin, 104
enzymes
    biotin-containing, 93
    digestive, 28, 119
    and enzymatic reactions, 120
    flavoprotein, 147
    fluoride and, 109
    liver, 106, 118, 128
    manganese and, 123
    and zinc, 165, 166
epilepsy, 123
epithelial tissue, 142, 143
esomeprazole, 23
estrogen, 94, 95
    conjugated and esterified, 110, 120, 148, 151
    gene expression, 152
estrogen replacement therapy (ERT), 73–75. See also female hormones; oral contraceptives
ethacrynic acid, 16, 95, 120, 131, 144, 151, 156, 165
ethambutol, 6, 106
    mineral depletions caused by, 30, 165
ethsuximide, 110
etodolac, 110
extracellular
    electrolytes, 138
    fluids, 99
eye problems
    vitamin A and, 142, 143
    vitamin B_2, 147
    vitamin E and, 162, 163
    zinc and, 166

fainting, 34
famotidine, 23, 95, 110, 116, 154, 159, 165
fatigue
    as drug effect, 26, 27, 34
    as effect of nutrient deficiency, 94, 102, 106, 111, 114, 117, 121, 131, 143, 145, 155, 163
fatty acids, 92, 117, 123, 124, 145, 150, 162. See also metabolism
Fe^{+++} and Fe^{++}, 117
fear (magnesium deficiency symptom), 121
felodipine, 15
female hormones, 19, 69
fenofibrate, 18, 67, 104, 106, 161, 165
fenoprofen, 110
fiber, dietary, 91
fibrates, 18, 67
5-HTP, 134
flavins, 146, 147
fluoride, 108
fluoroquinolones, 91, 92, 113, 118, 144, 146, 148, 151, 154, 164
fluorosis, 109–110
fluphenazine, 21, 104, 146
fluvastatin, 17, 104
folic acid (folacin)
    depletion, 26, 31, 63
    nutrient deficiency of, 110–113, 133, 155, 157
Folkers, Professor Karl, 104
foscarnet, 12, 56, 120, 131
fosinopril, 14, 165
fosphenytoin, 95, 110, 159, 164
free radicals, 90, 105, 125, 127, 133, 135, 158, 162, 163, 166
furosemide, 16, 95, 120, 131, 144, 151, 156, 165

GABA, 153
gait, abnormal/stumbling, 153, 155
"garlicky" breath, 136
gastric ulcers, 109
gastrointestinal distress, 26. See also intestinal system and disorders
gemfibrozil, 18, 68, 104, 161
gene expression, 167
genetic code, 155
gentamicin, 5, 33
gingivitis, 105, 143
glimepride, 104
glucose and glucose metabolism, 98, 123, 141, 145, 153, 159
glucose tolerance factor (GTF), 102, 103, 149
glutathione, 133, 133, 147
glutathione perioxidase, 135
glyburide, 9, 104
glycogen, 141, 153
glycoproteins, 124
goiter, 114, 116

goitrogens, 115
gout, 159
gout medications, 20, 75–76
gouty arthritis, 127
growth
  factor, 154
  hormone, 126
  zinc and, 167

H-2 blockers (H-2 receptor antagonists), 23,
  80–82
hair health and loss, 26, 93, 99, 106, 111,
  117, 136, 147, 162, 166
hallucinations, 155
haloperidol, 22, 79, 104, 125, 161
HDL cholesterol, 103, 149, 158
headache
  as drug effect, 17, 26
  migraine, 109
  and nutrient depletion, 111, 126, 143, 163
healing
  vitamin C and, 158
  zinc and, 166, 167
*The Healing Factor: Vitamin C Against
  Disease*, 156
Health LifeLine, x
hearing loss, 37, 160
heart
  attacks, 121, 122, 128, 135, 149
  calcium role in, 96
  carnitine and, 98
  coenzyme Q_{10} and, 105
  irregularities, 34, 93
  palpitation, 26, 96
  potassium role in, 27, 131
  vitamin B_1 and, 145
Helicobacter pylori, 80–81
hemochromatosis, 118
hemoglobin, 107, 116, 117, 151, 153
hemorrhage, 37, 157
heparin, 139
hepatitis, 134
hexuronic acid, 156
histamines, 149, 153, 157
HMG-COA reductase inhibitors, 17, 66
homocysteine, 26, 33, 111, 112, 133,
  152, 153
hormone replacement therapy (HRT), 73.
  See also oral contraceptives
hot flashes, 162
hyaluronidase, 157
hydralazine, 104, 151
hydralazine-containing vasodilators, 16, 60–61
hydrochloric acid, 100
hydrochlorothiazide (HCTZ), 16, 95, 104,
  120, 131, 165
hydroflumethiazide, 104, 110, 120, 131, 138,
  165
hydrogen peroxide, 119, 135

hydroxyapitite, 96
hydroxychloroquine, 33
hydroxylation reactions, 94
hydroxyzine, 9, 48–49, 125
hyperbilirubinaemia, 134
hypercalcemia, 161
hyperkalemia, 132
hypertension, 26, 97, 121, 122, 132
hyperthyroidism, 130
hypervitaminosis A, 143
hypochlorhydria, 117
hypocholesterolemia, 123
hypoglycemia, 103, 123, 128
hypotension, 34
hypothyroidism, 114
hysterectomies, 112

ibuprofen, 11, 110
imipramine, 21, 104, 146
immune system, xii
  beta-carotene and, 90
  bifidobacteria bifidum, and, 91
  CoQ_{10} and, 105
  fluoride and, 109
  iron and, 117, 119
  L. acidophilus and, 119
  selenium and, 134, 135
  vitamin D and, 161
  vitamin E and, 163
  zinc and, 167
immunity, 142
  vitamin C and, 158
  zinc and, 166
indapamide, 16, 104, 120, 131, 138, 165
indigestion, antacids for, 27
indomethacin, 11, 53, 110, 116, 156
infants, premature, 162
infections
  frequency of and susceptibility to, 26, 106,
    111, 117, 163, 166
  opportunistic, 55, 56
inositol, 113–114, 149
insomnia, 121
  antacids and, 26
  calcium deficiency and, 96
  folic acid deficiency and, 111
  as isoniazid effect, 29–30
  melatonin deficiency and, 27, 125
  vitamin B_3 deficiency and, 29
  vitamin B_6 deficiency and, 152
insulin, 102, 103, 105, 123, 128, 139, 140,
  149, 167
interferon, 158
intestinal system and disorders, 91, 121, 130,
  145, 146, 148
intracellular fluids, 99, 131
intramuscular injection, 156
intrinsic factor, 81, 154, 155
iodine, 114–116

iron, 107, 116–118, 157
  depletion from antibiotics, 34
  supplementation, 53, 82
  toxicity, 118
irregular heartbeat, 131
irritability, 121
islets of Langerhans, 78
isoniazid (IHH), 6, 29–30, 148, 151, 159

joints, 139, 139
  pain, 157, 166
Journal of the American Medical Association
  (JAMA), xii

kanamycin, 5, 33
keratin, 139
keratinization, 143
ketones, 98
ketoprofen, 110
kidney
  diseases, 121, 166, 109
  malfunction/failure, 130, 131, 132, 160
  stones, 121, 159
knock-knees, 160
Krebs cycle, 149, 150

labored breathing, 117
lactation, nutritional needs during, 96, 113
lactic acid, 119
Lactobacillus acidophilus, 28, 91, 118–120
lactose intolerance, 97, 145
lamivudine, 98, 106
lansoprazole, 23, 154
laxatives, 20–22
LDL cholesterol, 103, 105, 149, 158, 162
L-dopa/levodopa, 11, 54, 131, 132, 151
lean body mass, 103
lecithin, 101
lethargy, 152, 167
levothyroxine, 23, 80, 116
lipid
  metabolism, 102
  peroxidation, 135
lipoic acid, 140
lipopolysaccharides, 124
lipoprotein(a) (Lp(a)), 158
lipoprotein lipase, 141
lipotrophic agent, 101
lisinopril, 14, 165
lithium, 22, 79
liver
  detoxification, 133
  diseases, 121, 133, 150
  function, 98, 101, 106, 118, 126, 128, 140, 160
  vitamin A in, 142
  vitamin B_{12} in, 154
  vitamin D and, 160
  vitamin K and, 164
  zinc and, 166, 167

loop diuretics, 16, 61–63, 138
lovostatin, 17, 104
lymphocytes. *See* white blood cells
lysine, 98

macrocytic anemia, 155
macrolides, 91, 92, 113, 118, 144, 146, 148,
  151, 154, 164
macrophages, 161
macular degeneration, 166
magnesium, 31, 35, 94, 95, 96, 120–123, 140
magnesium/aluminum hydroxide antacids, 26
magnesium-containing antacids, 110
malnutrition vomiting, 131
manganese, 123–124
MAO inhibitors, 134
McCully, Dr. Kilmer, x
mefenamic acid, 11
megaloblastic anemia, 111
melanin, 107, 124
melatonin, 27, 30, 125–126, 152
memory loss, 138, 145, 145, 155
Menkes' disease, 107
menopause. *See* female hormones; oral
  contraceptives
menstruation. *See also* PMS
  loss of iron and, 116
  zinc deficiency and, 166
mental confusion/disturbances, 126, 131, 132
mercury, 135
mesoridazine, 21, 104, 146
metabolic alkalosis, 99
metabolism, 45, 74, 75, 94, 128
  bone, 108, 166
  calcium, 94, 96, 122
  of carbohydrates, 93, 122, 147, 149, 150,
    155
  fat, 98, 101, 117, 147, 149, 150, 155
  of folic acid, 155
  glucose, 123, 141
  phosphorus and, 129
  protein/amino acid, 93, 97, 102, 122, 123,
    127, 149, 150, 151, 152, 153, 155
  tyrosine, 157
  vitamin B_{12} and, 154
metabolites, 160
metformin, 8, 104, 110, 154
methdilazine, 146
methionine, 30, 57, 61, 98, 112, 132, 133,
  139, 152, 155
methotrexate, 24, 83, 110
methotrimeprazine, 146
methyclothiazide, 104, 165
methyldopa, 15, 60, 104
methylprednisolone, 10
metolazone, 16, 104, 120, 131, 165
metoprolol, 125
microflora, 28, 34
micronutrients, 97

mineral(s), xii
  ascorbates, 159
  trace, 94, 102, 106, 126, 134, 136, 140
mineralization, 137, 161
mineral oil, 20, 76, 90, 95, 142, 159, 161, 164
mitochondria, 98, 105, 147
mitochondrial superoxide dismutase, 124
mitral valve prolapse, 105
moexipril, 165
molybdenum, 126
monoamine oxidase inhibitors (MAOs), 22, 78–79
moodiness, 155
mucolytic agents, 115
mucopolysaccharides, 123, 123, 124, 137, 140
mucus membranes, inflamed, 146
muscle
  cramps, 26, 96, 121
  incoordination, 153, 167
  pain, 93
  weakness, 27, 34, 98, 131, 138, 157, 160, 162, 163
myelin and myelination, 133, 155
myoglobin, 117
myoinositol, 113, 114
myxedema, 115

NAD (nicotinamide adenine dinucleotide), 148, 149
nadolol, 14
NADP (nicotinamide adenine dinucleotide phosphate), 148, 149
NADPH oxidation, 141
naproxen, 11, 110
nausea
  as drug effect, 26
  as nutrient depletion effect, 93, 94, 111, 152, 155, 163
neomycin, 5, 33, 90, 116, 142, 154
nerve impulses and function, 132, 138
nervousness, 26, 115, 121
nervous system and disorders
  as drug effect, 26, 34
  from nutrient depletion, 96, 102, 106, 112, 131, 136, 145, 148, 150, 152, 155
neuromuscular system, 145
neuron regeneration, 133
neuropeptides, 133
neurotransmitters, 29, 57, 60, 100, 116, 118, 133, 145, 150, 153
Neutrophilic Hypersegmentation Index (NHI), 111
nevirapine, 98, 106, 154, 165
New Passages, xi
niacin, 103, 111, 148–150, 153
niacinamide, 149
niacin flush, 103, 149
nicardene, 15
nickel, 127–129

nickel carbonyl, 129
nickeloplasmin, 128
nicotinic acid, 149, 149
nifedipine, 15, 59, 131
night blindness, 142, 143, 166
nitrosamines, 157
nizatidine, 23, 95, 110, 116, 154, 159, 165
noradrenalin, 157
norepinephrine, 153, 157
nortriptyline, 21, 104, 146
NSAIDS (non-steroidal anti-inflammatory drugs), 11, 53–54, 110, 125
nucleic acids, 133
numbness, and nutrient deficiency, 93, 102, 132, 145
nutrient depletion, drug-induced, vii, ix
nutritional deficiency diseases, x
nutritional supplements, x–xii

omega-3 fatty acids, 41
omeprazole, 23, 154
opportunistic infections, 55, 56
oral contraceptives, 19, 69–75, 110, 120, 134, 144, 146, 148, 151, 153, 154, 156, 165
organidin, 115
orlistat, 90
osmotic equilibrium/pressure, 99, 132, 138
osteoarthritis, 137
osteocalcin, 164
osteomalacia, 26, 34, 96, 160, 164
osteoporosis, 26, 94, 96, 97, 107, 108, 109, 123, 130, 160, 161, 164
oxalates, 117
oxalic acid, 159
oxidases, 147
oxidation-reduction reactions, 147, 149, 157

pagophagia, 117
pain
  back, 26, 96
  leg, 26, 96
  muscle, 93
  of osteoporosis and osteomalacia, 38
pancreas, 78. See also insulin
pantoprazole, 23
pantotheine, 150
pantothenic acid, 150–151
para-aminosalicylic acid, 6, 33
parathyroid gland, 161
Parkinson's disease, 124
pellagra, 148
penicillamine, 24, 84–85, 106, 107, 116, 120, 151, 165
penicillin antibiotics, 5, 34, 91, 92, 113, 118, 131, 144, 146, 148, 151, 154, 164
pentamidine, 11, 55, 120
periodontal disease, 105
peripheral neuropathy, 155

pernicious anemia, 154, 155
perphenazine, 104, 146
perspiration, sodium and, 138
pH. *See* acid/alkaline
phenelzine, 22, 78–79, 151
phenobarbital, 7, 38, 92, 95, 110, 151, 159, 164
phenothiazines, 21, 78
phenytoin, 7, 38, 92, 95, 110, 144, 154, 159, 164
phosphate
  depletion, 26
  enemas, 21
phosphates/phosphorus, 26, 117
phosphatidylcholine (PC), 130, 133
phosphatidylinositol, 113
phosphodiesterase inhibitor, 158
phospholipids, 101, 113, 114, 130, 133, 150
phosphoric acid, 130, 145, 147
phosphorus, 96, 129, 160, 161
photophobia, 166
phytates, 117
phytic acid, 113, 114
pigeon breast, 160
pindolol, 14
pineal gland, 125
piroxicam, 11
pituitary, 99, 114, 123, 131
platelet aggregation/stickiness, 121, 122, 162
PMS, 43, 122, 152, 153, 162, 163
polyamines, 133
polythiazide, 104, 120, 131, 165
porphyrin, 150
potassium, 34, 131–132
potassium chloride, 18, 34, 68–69, 154
potassium-sparing diuretics, 16, 63–64
pravastatin, 17, 104
prednisone, 10
pregnancy
  calcium needs during, 96
  folic acid needs during, 32, 111, 113
  iodine deficiency during, 115
  vitamin A during, 144
  vitamin B$_2$ and, 148
  zinc needs during, 166
primidone, 8, 43, 92, 110
probenicid, 90
probiotics, 28, 29, 34, 35, 91–92, 119, 120
prochlorperazine, 104, 146
promazine, 104, 146
promethazine, 104, 146
propranolol, 14, 58, 104, 104, 125
propstaglandins, 151, 158
protein, and protein metabolism, 75, 81, 93, 97, 102, 122, 123, 138, 147, 150, 157
protein calorie malnutrition, 135
prothrombin, 124, 164
proton pump inhibitors, 23, 80, 82–83
protriptyline, 104, 146

provitamin A, 90, 144. *See also* beta-carotene
psoriasis, 129, 161, 162
psychiatric disorders, 105, 148
psychotherapeutic drugs, 21–22, 77–79
pteroylmonoglutamate, 111
puescine, 133
pyridine nucleotides, 148
pyridoxal phosphate (PLP), 151, 153
pyridoxine, 151–154. *See also* vitamin B$_6$

quinapril, 14
quinestrol, 120, 151
quinethazone, 104, 120, 131, 165
quinines, 164

raberprazole, 23
ramipril, 14, 165
ranitidine, 23, 95, 110, 116, 154, 159, 165
Recommended Dietary Allowance (RDAs), x, xi, xii
red blood cells, 155
reflexes, poor, 27, 34, 131
reserpine, 104
restlessness, 121
retinoids, 142
retinol. *See* vitamin A
retinol equivalents (R.E.), 144
reverse transcriptase inhibitors, 55–56
rheumatic pain, 160
riboflavin, 146–148
rickets, 96, 160, 164
rifampin, and vitamin D, 6, 30–31, 159
ritodrine, 24, 85, 131
RNA, 112, 120, 128, 130, 155, 167
rosuvastatin calcium, 17

s-adenosyl methionine (SAME), 132–134
salicylates, 10, 52–53, 116, 138, 150
salsalate, 11, 110
salt, 100, 131, 138, 139. *See also* sodium chloride
  iodized, 116
  –taste perception, and zinc, 167
schizophrenia, 123, 124
scientific basis, viii–ix
scurvy, 156, 157
seborrheic dermatitis, 152
selective serotonin reuptake inhibitors (SSRIs), 22, 79
selenium, 134–136, 162
sensory perceptions, zinc and, 17
serotonin, 29, 30, 57, 60, 74, 118, 125, 151, 152, 153, 157
serum cholesterol, 30
Sheehy, Gail, xi
side-effects, vii
silicon, 136
silicosis, 137
simvastatin, 17, 104

skeletal abnormalities, 26, 123, 137
skin
  copper depletion and, 106
  dry, scaly, and beta-carotene deficiency, 90
  pallor, 117
  rashes and boron deficiency, 94
  silicon and, 137
  vitamins and, 29, 147, 148, 150, 162
  zinc and, 166
sleep, melatonin and, 125
sodium, 138–139
sodium ascorbate, 158
sodium bicarbonate, 4, 27, 131
sodium bicarbonate antacids, 26–27
sodium chloride (salt), 99
sodium phosphate enema, 21
sodium/potassium pump, 138
sotolol, 14
spermidine, 133
spinal curvature, 160
spooning (fingernail), 117
SSKI, 115
SSRIs (selective serotonin reuptake inhibitors), 22, 138
stanozolol, 22, 79–80, 116
starvation, 138
statin drugs, 66
stavudine, 98, 106
sterility, 162
steroid(s)
  anabolic, 22, 79–80
  hormones, 150
Stone, Irwin, 156
streptomycin, 5, 33
stress
  and intestinal distress, 91
  potassium deficiency and, 131
  vitamin C and, 157
strokes, 105, 121, 128, 132, 135
sucralfate, 95
sugar, 102, 131
sulfasalazine, 11, 53, 110
sulfate, 126
sulfhydryl, 140
sulfite oxidase, 127
sulfolipids, 140
sulfonamides, 91, 92, 113, 118, 144, 146, 148, 151, 154, 164
sulfonylureas, 9, 46
sulfur, 139–140
sulfuric acid, 140
sulindac, 11
sunlight, vitamin D and, 160, 161
sweating, and nutrient deficiency, 99
Szent–Gyorgy, Albert, xii, 156

tachycardia, 115, 126
tardive dyskinesia, 101
taurine, 133, 139

teeth
  calcium role in, 96
  decay as drug effect, 26
  fluoride and, 108
  magnesium and, 120, 122
  silicon and, 137
  vanadium and, 141
  vitamins and, 143, 157, 160
terbutaline, 13, 131
testosterone, 94
tetany, 34
tetracycline antibiotics, 5, 34, 91, 92, 95, 113, 116, 118, 120, 144, 146, 148, 151, 154, 156, 164, 165
tetrahydrofolic acid, (THFA), 111
theophylline-containing drugs, 13, 56–57, 151
thiamin, 139, 140, 144
thiamin pyrophosphate (TPP), 145
thiazide diuretics, 16, 64–65, 138
thiethylperazine, 104
thioridazine, 21, 104, 146
thirst, continuous, 34, 131
thrombus, 74
thymus, 150
thyroid
  hormones, 114, 115, 135
  medications, 23, 80
thyroid-releasing hormone (TRH), 114
thyroid-stimulating hormone, 114
thyroxin, 124, 157, 167
timolol, 14
tingling in hands and feet, 153
T-lymphocytes, 135
tobramycin, 5, 33
tocopherol. See alpha tocopherol
tolazamide, 9, 104
tolbutamide, 104
torsemide, 95, 120, 131, 144, 151, 156, 165
total parenteral nutrition (TPN), 126
toxins, metal, 135, 158
trace minerals, xii, 94, 102, 106, 126, 134, 136, 140
trandolapril, 14, 165
transamination, 153
transsulfuration, 133
triamcinolone, 10
triamterene, 16, 63, 64, 95, 110, 110, 165
trichlomethiazide, 104, 120, 131, 165
trifluoperazine, 146
trimethoprim, 35, 144, 146, 148, 151, 154, 164
tricyclic antidepressants, 21, 77–78
trifluoperazine, 104
triglycerides, 102, 141
triiodothyronine, 135, 167
trimethoprim, 6, 35, 92, 110, 113
trimethylamine, 101
trimipramine, 104, 146
tryptophan, 29, 57, 60, 72, 134, 148, 149, 150, 152, 153

tuberculosis-treating ... scorbic acid), 111, 156–159
tyrosine, 72, 157 ... alciferol), 30, 33, 94, 96, 122,
159–161

ubiquinone, 104
ulcer medications, 80
ultraviolet rays, 160, 161
"uncombable hair syndrome," 93
uric acid, 127
U.S. Department of Agriculture survey on
  magnesium, 120
U.S. Environmental Protection Agency,
  suggested range for fluoride in municipal
  water supplies, 110

valproic acid, 8, 45, 98, 106, 110, 134, 165
vanadium, 140–142
vasodilators and vasodilation, 60–61, 149
vegetarians
  iron and, 116
  vitamin B$_{12}$ and, 155
verapamil, 15, 59, 131
viruses, vitamin C and, 158
vision, and vitamin A, 143
vitamin A (retinol), 90, 142–144, 167
vitamin B$_1$ (thiamin), 144–146
vitamin B$_2$ (riboflavin), 146–148
vitamin B$_3$ (niacin), 29, 31, 148–150
vitamin B$_5$ (pantothenic acid), 150
vitamin B$_6$ (pyridoxine), 29, 31, 125, 151–154
vitamin B$_{12}$ (cyanocobalamin), 31, 33, 133,
  154–156

vitamin E (alpha tocopherol)., 117, 158,
  161–163
vitamin K, 31, 119, 124, 164–165
vomiting, 99, 138, 152, 155, 167

weakness,
  as drug effect, 27
  and nutrient deficiency, 98, 117, 121, 131,
    138, 157, 160, 162, 163
weight gain
  and chromium deficiency, 102
  and iodine deficiency, 114
weight-loss, 98
wellness, x
Wernicke-Korsakoff syndrome, 145
white blood cells, 158
Williams, Dr. Roger, 150
Wilson's disease, 107

xanthine oxidase, 97, 127
xerophthalmia, 142, 143

zalcitabine, 98
zidovudine (AZT), 12, 55–56, 98, 106, 154,
  165
zinc, 35, 106, 107, 165–168
zinc oxide, 167
zonisamide, 95, 110, 113, 144

DATE DUE
